How to Prevent or Even Reverse HEART DISEASE Without Drugs or Surgery!

By Robert D. Willix, Jr., M.D., FACSM

Notice: All material in this publication is provided for information only and may not be construed as medical advice or instruction. No action or inaction should be taken based solely on the contents of this publication; instead, readers should consult appropriate health professionals on any matter relating to their health and well-being. The information and opinions provided in this publication are believed to be accurate and sound, based on the best judgment available to the author, and readers who fail to consult with appropriate health authorities assume the risk of any injuries. Neither the publisher, the editors, nor the writers will be responsible for errors or ommissions, negligent or otherwise.

Copyright © 2005 by 1st Start Publishing, Inc.

All rights reserved. No part of this publication may be reproduced or transmitted in any form or by any means, electronic or mechanical, including photocopying, recording, or by any information storage and retrieval system, without permission in writing from the publishers.

Printed in the United States of America

Published by:
    1st Start Publishing, Inc.
    245 N.E. 4th Avenue
    Suite 201
    Delray Beach, Florida 33483

ISBN 0-9763613-0-2 softcover

Table of Contents

Introduction. 4

CHAPTER 1 6
What is Heart Disease?

CHAPTER 2 20
A Closer Look

CHAPTER 3 25
In the Doctor's Office

CHAPTER 4 48
Heart Healthy Eating

CHAPTER 5 90
The Exercise Factor

CHAPTER 6 104
Lifestyle Choices for a Healthy Heart

CHAPTER 7 115
Dietary Supplements for Heart Health

CHAPTER 8 135
How Herbs Can Help

CHAPTER 9 150
Natural Alternatives to Surgery

CHAPTER 10 162
How Complimentary Medicine Keeps You Young At Heart

About the Author 177

APPENDIX I. Resources 179

APPENDIX II. Glossary. 184

SELECTED REFERENCES 191

INTRODUCTION

If you've been the victim of a heart attack – or know someone who is – you know that life afterwards is forever changed. A victim of cardiovascular disease (CVD) lives in fear of when the next attack might strike. And if you haven't been stricken yet, count your blessings – because in the United States alone:

■ Nearly 62 million adults have one or more types of cardiovascular disease.

■ More than 2,500 people die from heart disease every day.

■ One person suffers a heart attack every 20 seconds.

■ Despite new conventional treatments, cardiovascular disease is on the rise.

Of all the deaths in the United States each year, cardiovascular disease causes more than 40 percent. Many of these people were under the age of 65 – and more than half were women. The sad truth, as you can see from the graph below, is that cardiovascular disease (CVD) is the No. 1 killer in America – more than cancer, diabetes or even accidents.

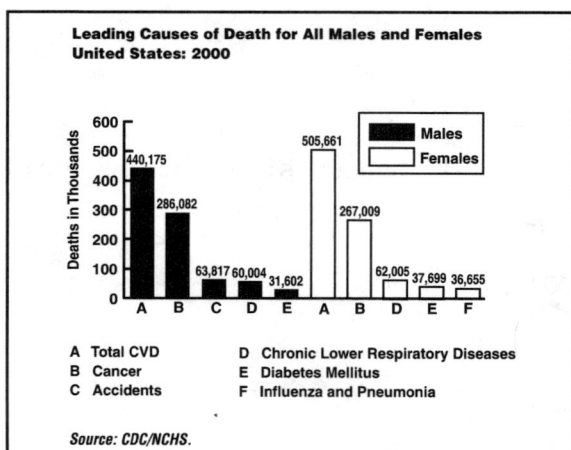

Leading Causes of Death for All Males and Females United States: 2000

Deaths in Thousands

Males
Females

A: 440,175 | B: 286,082 | C: 63,817 | D: 60,004 | E: 31,602
A: 505,661 | B: 267,009 | D: 62,005 | E: 37,699 | F: 36,655

A Total CVD
B Cancer
C Accidents
D Chronic Lower Respiratory Diseases
E Diabetes Mellitus
F Influenza and Pneumonia

Source: CDC/NCHS.

As a former cardiac surgeon, these statistics are indeed disturbing. I believe that the reason behind these staggering numbers is that conventional medicine, spurred on by the pharmaceutical industry, has only focused its attention on part of the problem – cholesterol. But, despite what your doctor may tell you, high cholesterol levels aren't the most important factor in determining whether or not you'll develop this potentially deadly disease. Indeed, two other factors – high homocystine and C-reactive protein levels – are much better indicators.

There is also compelling scientific evidence that our lifestyle choices – diet, exercise, whether or not we smoke – can significantly increase the odds of developing heart disease. In the following pages, you'll learn how different, healthier choices can dramatically reduce or even prevent its occurrence. I'll also discuss the role modern medicine plays in heart disease and show you a number of safe, effective ways you can avoid costly, and potentially dangerous, surgery and drugs.

Many of the alternatives outlined in this book may be things you've never heard of – either from your doctor or the popular press. But they are things that can help you live longer, feel better and prevent or reverse heart disease. Best of all, you can start benefiting from many of these natural therapies right now. So let's get started!

Chapter 1

WHAT IS HEART DISEASE?

Your heart is a complex and magnificent organ. Although it only weighs between eight and fourteen ounces, this hollow muscle is responsible for circulating blood throughout your entire body. When it's working properly, a healthy heart beats 100,000 times a day. These rhythmic contractions send oxygen-rich blood and nutrients to the body's tissues. By the time you are seventy, your heart will beat nearly 2.6 billion times and pump some 35.8 million gallons of blood.

Your heart is divided into two halves, each designed to direct blood in one direction only. The right half receives the blood returning from every part of your body after the oxygen has been used by the tissues and organs. The right half then pumps this oxygen-deficient blood into your lungs through a vessel called the pulmonary artery. There, the blood picks up oxygen before traveling to the left half of your heart. Think of as the ultimate recycler.

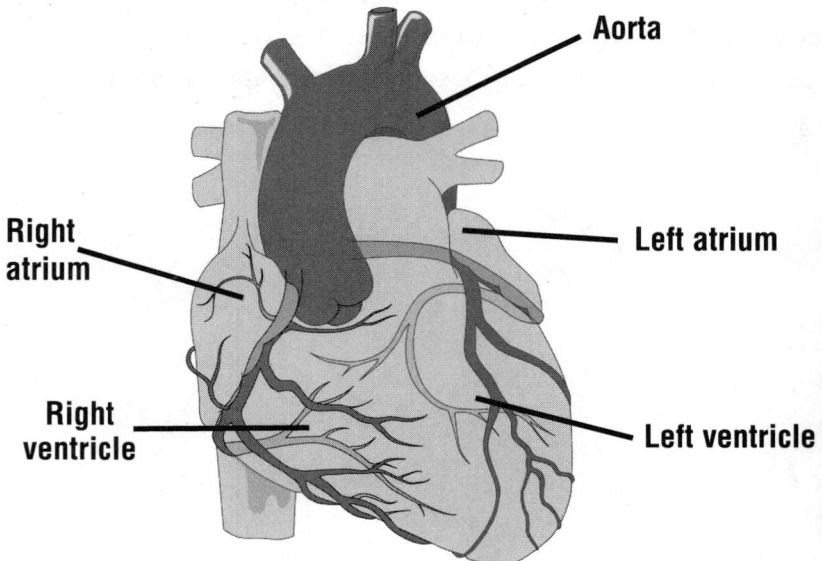

Once this newly oxygenated blood makes its way back to the left side of your heart, it is pumped into the aorta, the largest artery in your body. From there, the process starts all over again as the blood is sent to all of the other arteries in your body.

You may have guessed by now that a steady supply of oxygen is essential. Unlike other muscles in the body, which can function without oxygen, the heart depends on this vital gas to function properly. During the resting period between each heartbeat, the heart also supplies blood to itself, delivering oxygen and other critical nutrients that allow it to maintain its constant pumping action. In fact, the heart needs as much as a pint of blood per minute to work properly.

One of the most important reasons the heart needs this continual blood supply is to sustain its electrical activity. Every time your heart contracts, electrical impulses pass over its surface in a rhythmic pattern and are transformed into electromagnetic energy waves that travel through the heart's muscle cells. This is the same electrical energy that is detected during an electrocardiogram (EKG).

If your heart becomes stressed, it can form alternative routes to provide blood supply to the undernourished muscles by adjusting blood flow and the signals created by the nervous system. Your heart can also grow new blood vessels. The heart's amazing adaptability, however, depends on the health of its coronary arteries, which in turn depends on the health of each artery's inner lining.

This inner lining is made up of tissue called the endothelium. When this tissue is healthy, it maintains the normal tone of the blood vessels through its effect on the smooth muscles in the outer part of the vessel wall. The endothelium also plays an important role in controlling the stickiness of platelets (small cells in the blood). Although these platelets help stop bleeding when you cut yourself, they also cling to any tears in the blood vessels lining and can narrow the arteries.

How Arteries Become Clogged

Heart disease begins when plaque builds up and eventually narrows the arteries, a condition called *atherosclerosis*. Plaque is a fatty substance made up of cholesterol and other fats or lipids, calcium and a blood-clotting material called fibrin which causes the endothelium tissue to malfunction. In response, the endothelium releases a chemical that creates a sticky surface which attracts other cells. Over time, this build-up, known as atherosclerosis, narrows the arteries and causes blood flow to slow. Ultimately, this narrowing will prevent the heart from getting the oxygen and nutrients it needs to function properly.

A heart attack usually starts when this plaque ruptures and forms a dangerous blood clot. The clot may stay put or it may travel down an artery until it hits another obstructed area. If it does travel, it may block up to 95 percent of the blood flow. There may even be a complete blockage of the artery. Even though only 10 to 20 percent of the plaques in our body have a high probability of rupturing, they are responsible for 80 to 90 percent of all serious heart problems, including chest pain (angina) and heart attacks.

Many of the natural remedies in this book can improve endothelial cell function. Enhancing this function widens the blood vessels and reduces the chance that a sudden blockage will occur if a plaque bursts. In the next chapter, I'll give you a more detailed look at how plaque and atherosclerosis can lead to heart disease.

Are You At Risk?

There are a number of risk factors for heart disease. Unfortunately, some are beyond our control. For example, as we get older, our hearts don't work as efficiently. For much of our lives, gender also plays a role. Until a woman reaches menopause, men have a higher risk of a heart attack. But after menopause, a woman's risk actually triples! By the time a woman reaches the age of 65, her risk is almost equal to a man's.

Family history also plays its part. Most people with a strong family history of heart disease have one or more other risk factors. Just as you can't control your age or gender, you can't control your family history. Therefore, it's even more important to address the risk factors you can control:

- **Smoking**
- **Stress**
- **Inflammation**
- **Diabetes**
- **High Blood Pressure**
- **High Homocystine Levels**
- **High Cholesterol and Triglyceride Levels**
- **Sedentary Lifestyle**
- **Obesity**

Smoking: Kicking the cigarette habit is perhaps the single most important thing you can do to protect yourself against heart disease. Consider this:

√ Cigarette smoking is the biggest risk factor for sudden cardiac death.

√ Of the more than 400,000 Americans who die every year from smoking, the majority die from heart disease, not lung disease.

√ Cigarette smoking produces a greater risk for coronary heart disease in people younger than 50 years.

√ The American Heart Association estimates indicate that approximately 37,000 to 40,000 people die each year from heart and blood vessel disease caused by secondhand smoke.

Inhaling tobacco smoke causes several immediate responses within the heart and its blood vessels. Within one minute of starting to smoke, the heart rate begins to rise: it may increase by as much as 30 percent during the first 10 minutes of smoking. Nicotine raises blood pressure: blood vessels constrict which forces the heart to work harder to deliver oxygen to the rest of the body. Meanwhile, the carbon monoxide in tobacco smoke exerts a negative effect on the heart by reducing the blood's ability to carry oxygen.

Smoking also tends to increase cholesterol levels. In fact, the ratio of HDL to LDL cholesterol tends to be lower in smokers compared to non-smokers.   Cigarette smokers also have raised levels of fibrinogen (a protein which causes blood to clot) and platelets which make the blood stickier. Carbon monoxide attaches itself to hemoglobin (the oxygen-carrying pigment in red blood cells) much more easily than oxygen does. This reduces the amount of oxygen available to the tissues by forming compound called carboxy-hemoglobin, which is only present in the blood of smokers. All these factors make smokers more at risk of developing atherosclerosis.

If you smoke, quit. Yes, it's hard to do, but it's well worth it. Researchers from the World Health Organization say that a smoker's risk of having a heart attack is slashed by 50 percent after only of year of quitting.

Stress: While it's difficult to document the effects of stress on heart disease, it is clear that constant stress has a very negative effect. Researchers have found that stress triggers a number of physiological changes that affect the heart. Stress causes the adrenal glands to release epinephrine, better known as adrenaline, which makes the heart pump faster and the lungs work harder to flood the body with oxygen. The adrenal glands also release the hormone cortisol, which helps the body convert sugar to energy. While this is a normal reaction to short-term stress, when stress becomes an all-day, every-day occurrence, this constant flood of hormones can raise your blood pressure and damage the lining of your arteries, making it a prime target for plaque build-up. Blood clots are also more likely to form during times of stress and could block an already-narrowed artery. Fortunately, there are a number of ways to reduce stress – many of which I discuss in Chapter 7.

Inflammation: Inflammation is now recognized as an important contributing factor to atherosclerosis and heart disease. While short bouts of inflammation help the body heal itself from injury or infection, long-term episodes of inflammation within the arteries can do great damage. It seems that plaque is naturally drawn to the site of inflammation and, as the years pass, layer after layer is deposited inside the artery, eventually causing many of the symptoms of cardiovascular disease, including strokes and heart attacks.

One of the best ways to determine inflammation is by measuring C-reactive protein, or CRP. CRP is produced in the liver and is a strong predictor of a first-time heart attack, even in cases where cholesterol levels are normal. In one study, Harvard researchers reviewed the data from 1,086 men participating in the Physicians' Health Study – half of whom had experienced a heart attack, stroke or blood clot in a major vessel and half who had not. After analyzing the data, the Harvard team found that the men with the highest CRP levels were three times more likely to suffer a heart attack and twice as likely to have a stroke than the subjects with normal levels.

Other studies have also detected CRP in atherosclerotic lesions, where it has been found to attract white blood cells called monocytes and increase the production of sticky molecules in endothelial cells. Because the emerging research is so compelling, doctors should routinely test CRP levels as part of the battery of blood tests used for determining cardiovascular risk. CRP levels in the blood are normally undetectable or very low; levels greater than 2.0 are strongly associated with inflammation. Blood CRP, homocystine, and lipids (cholesterol and triglycerides) should be tested at least once a year.

Diabetes: Diabetes poses a major threat to your cardiovascular system, putting you at increased risk of having a heart attack or stroke. In fact, after analyzing data collected from two large multi-center clinical trials, Duke University Medical Center researchers found that patients with diabetes have almost twice the risk of dying or suffering severe outcomes from heart disease compared to non-diabetics.

Chronic high blood sugar is associated with the narrowing of the arteries, increased blood levels of triglycerides, decreased levels of "good" HDL cholesterol, high blood pressure and heart attack. While managing diabetes can reverse these effects, the symptoms of diabetes can often go unnoticed.

People who are unaware that they have diabetes face an increased risk for heart disease because atherosclerosis may occur at an earlier age and may cause what is called "silent ischemia" or a silent heart attack. Silent, in this case, means without typical pain because neuropathy, or nerve damage, is a result of uncontrolled diabetes.

High Blood Pressure: High blood pressure is a condition that occurs when the pressure inside your large arteries is too high. Also known as hypertension, high blood pressure is the first step in the quiet decent towards heart disease and stroke. In fact, according to the American Heart Association, high blood pressure was directly linked to 44,435 deaths in 1998 and indirectly responsible for another 210,000 deaths.

Since high blood pressure rarely shows any symptoms, unless your doctor monitors your blood pressure on a regular basis, it's easy to miss — until it's too late. A 50-year study by the National Heart, Lung and Blood Institute (NHLBI), known as the Framingham Heart Study, found that half of all people who have suffered a first heart attack also had moderate to high blood pressure.

Normal blood pressure is approximately 119/80 millimeters of mercury or below. Blood pressure naturally goes up as you age and the arteries become less elastic. When blood pressure reaches 140/90 or above on a consistent basis, you have high blood pressure. While aging can cause your blood pressure to rise, obesity, heavy alcohol use, high salt intake, a sedentary lifestyle and stress can also cause hypertension. Fortunately, these factors are something you can control.

Homocystine: Homocystine is the normal breakdown product of the essential amino acid, methionine. Although the body uses small amounts of homocystine, high levels in the blood can boost LDL cholesterol levels. Homocystine also irritates the arteries and makes the blood clot more easily than it should, increasing the risk of blood vessel blockages. To make matters worse, homocystine prevents the small arteries from dilating so they are more vulnerable to obstruction.

Although conventional medicine ignored homocystine for decades, recent research has found a definite link between heart disease and high homocystine levels. In one study of 21,500 men, those with the highest homocystine levels were three times more likely to die of ischemic heart disease. *Silence the sign of pain*

How much is too much? A growing number of studies show that a homocystine level greater than 9 μmol/L is a risk factor for heart disease independent of other known risk factors such as high serum cholesterol. According to the *New England Journal of Medicine*, a four and a half year examination of the relationship between plasma homocystine and mortality was carried out by Norwegian researchers in 587 patients with coronary artery disease. Of the 64 patients who died during the study, only 3.8 percent of those whose plasma homocystine was less than 9 μmol/L died, compared with 25 percent of those with plasma homocystine above 15 μmol/L.

Mortality over four years in 587 patients with coronary artery disease	
Homocystine (μmol/L)	*Mortality (%)*
<9	*3.8*
9-14.9	*8.6*
≥15	*24.7*

Elevated homocystine levels can be caused by genetic enzyme deficiencies, dietary deficiencies of folic acid and vitamins B6 and B12, hypothyroidism or certain medications. For example, glucophage, used to treat diabetes, and cholestyramine, used to treat high triglycerides, block the absorption of folic acid from the intestines and raise blood levels of homocystine. Lifestyle factors also play a role, since cigarette smoking and caffeine can increase your homocystine levels. Unfortunately, homocystine levels also rise naturally as you get older. But, as you'll learn in Chapter 7, simply boosting your vitamin B and folic acid intake can dramatically lower homocystine levels.

High Cholesterol/High Triglyceride Levels: Cholesterol, a wax-like fatty substance that is produced in the liver, has gained a reputation as the primary risk factor for heart disease. But cholesterol isn't necessarily bad. In fact, our bodies need cholesterol to form cell membranes and to make sex and steroidal hormones, including estrogen, testosterone and cortisol. The trouble begins when we have too much of the wrong cholesterol.

Low-density lipoproteins (LDLs) are often called "bad" cholesterol because they carry cholesterol into the arteries, where it sticks to arterial walls and contributes to plaque build-up. High-density lipoproteins (HDLs), on the other hand, carry cholesterol out of the arteries and are known as "good" cholesterol. What really matters is the ratio of LDL to HDL. Scientific evidence suggests that LDL levels should not exceed HDL levels by more than four to five times. For example, if HDL levels are 60 mg/dL and LDL are 180 mg/dL, or three times greater than HDL, cholesterol is within an acceptable range.

While a poor ratio between LDL and HDL cholesterol can indeed boost your risk for heart disease, new evidence shows that it may not be the most important factor. The level of cholesterol in the blood provides a clue that something is wrong, nothing more.

Cholesterol doesn't travel around the bloodstream by itself. It is usually packaged with fats called triglycerides. Triglycerides are the body's preferred form of energy storage and usually come from the foods we eat. The calories that aren't immediately used by the tissues are converted to triglycerides and transported to fat cells to be stored. Hormones regulate the release of triglycerides from fat tissue so they meet the body's needs for energy between meals. But high levels of plasma triglycerides, a condition called hypertriglyceridemia, damages the arteries and increases your risk of atherosclerosis. People with high triglycerides often have high LDL and low HDL levels – a combination that is particularly dangerous. Chapter 4 provides more information on how to lower both cholesterol and triglyceride levels.

Sedentary Lifestyle: The old saying, "move it or lose it," certainly applies when it comes to heart disease. Yet, a shocking 24 percent of all Americans simply won't exercise – and if they do get the urge to work out, they simply wait until it passes.

Even moderate amounts of physical activity can reduce your risk of heart disease. Not only will you lower your weight and get your blood pumping – as you build muscle, you rev up your metabolism, causing your body to burn more fat and sugar for energy. This reduces your blood pressure and the levels of sugar and fat in the blood. In Chapter 6, we'll look at ways to fit heart-healthy exercise into your life.

Obesity: A healthy weight is crucial for a long, healthy life. Yet, in 1999, almost 61 percent of adults were overweight or obese. Being overweight dramatically increases your risk of heart attack. It also increases your risk of developing high blood cholesterol, high blood pressure and diabetes - each of which also increases your chance of having a heart attack. What's more, when you are obese, the wall of the heart must grow to be able to pump the additional blood volume required by your body. This makes the heart less efficient. And people who carry their weight around their waists are at an even higher risk, even if they have no other risk factors.

The easiest way to figure out if you have crossed the line from pleasantly plump to obese is to calculate your body mass index (BMI). Simply multiply your weight in pounds by 704.5. Then multiply your height in inches by your height in inches, and divide the first answer by the second answer. For example, if you are 5 feet, 8 inches and weigh 150 pounds:

$$150 \times 704.5 = 105,675$$
$$68 \times 68 = 4,624$$
$$105,675 \text{ divided by } 4,624 = 22.8$$

If you'd rather not do the math, there are a number of BMI calculators available on the internet. Just punch in your weight and height and – abracadabra! – your BMI is automatically calculated. What do the numbers mean? A BMI between 19 and 24 is considered normal. A BMI of 25 to 29 means you are overweight. And a reading of 30 or more indicates obesity.

Admittedly, losing weight can be a tough proposition. But, here's the good news: If you are overweight or obese, even a small loss – just 10 percent of your current weight – will help to lower your risk of developing heart disease.

A Word About Syndrome X

Syndrome X refers to a cluster of diet-related health problems that affect as many as 60 million Americans. Unfortunately, many of us are all too familiar with the signs of Syndrome X: that "spare tire" around the middle, high blood pressure, high triglycerides, high cholesterol levels. Although heart disease can be caused by any one of these risk factors, Syndrome X increases the probability of developing heart disease.

People who have Syndrome X do not respond well to insulin; they are insulin resistant. Their pancreas is forced to secrete excessive amounts of the insulin to dispose of glucose, or blood sugar, by moving it into muscles and fat cells. These people don't have diabetes, because they produce enough insulin to overcome the resistance, but the high insulin levels lead to elevated blood triglycerides (fatty acids), low HDL ("good") cholesterol, high blood pressure and other signs of Syndrome X.

HEART SMART TIP
IF YOU THINK YOU'RE INSULIN RESISTANT:

Ask your doctor for a hemoglobin A1C test. Unlike a glucose tolerance test, which simply measures the fluctuating blood sugar levels on a day-to-day basis, an A1C gives you an average of your blood sugar over the last three months.

As a baseball fan, I like to think of hemoglobin A1C as a way to figure your season batting average. A score of less than six means you're having a terrific season. Ratings over six, however, are diabetic ranges that can spell trouble.

In one study by researchers at Stanford University, 147 individuals (average age 50 and healthy at the start) were followed for five years. After reviewing the data, the researchers found that one out of seven of the subjects with the most insulin resistance had a heart attack during the study. But in those who were the least insulin resistant, not a single person had a heart attack.

Are you at risk for Syndrome X? If you are more than 15 pounds overweight, carry your weight around your middle, have high blood pressure, high triglycerides or low HDL levels, you might want to have a fasting blood glucose test and a glucose tolerance test. If your fasting

Normal insulin sensitivity levels:

Fasting — less than 20

After 1 hour — less than 80

After 2 hours — less than 60

After 3 hours — less than 40

glucose is more than 100 mg/dl and your glucose tolerance results are higher than 140 mg/dl, there is a good chance you are insulin resistant and may suffer from Syndrome X.

That said, I believe that insulin tolerance tests are much better than glucose tolerance tests for diagnosing Syndrome X. The test measures insulin sensitivity after the patient is given glucose (sugar). The box at the right lists the levels for someone who doesn't suffer from insulin resistance. But don't panic if your numbers are higher than those listed. This metabolic condition responds well to the diet, exercise and nutritional supplement advice outlined in this book.

REMEMBER . . .

➤ The heart can adapt to stress by adjusting blood flow and electrical activity, and by growing new blood vessels. But, even though your heart can make these adjustments, it can only do so if the coronary arteries are healthy.

➤ Heart disease begins when plaque builds up inside the arteries and eventually narrows them.

➤ A family history of heart disease and age are two risk factors beyond our control. But there are a number of risk factors you can control.

➤ Smoking is the most damaging contributor to heart disease. Quit now!

➤ CRP has recently been identified as a major risk factor for heart attack and stroke. Make sure your CRP levels are tested at least once a year.

➤ Your diet can contribute to diabetes, high blood pressure, high homocystine, unhealthy cholesterol levels and obesity – all risk factors for heart disease.

➤ Syndrome X, a cluster of diet-related health problems, also increases the chance of developing heart disease.

Chapter 2
A CLOSER LOOK

The term "heart disease" or "cardiovascular disease" covers a variety of heart-related conditions, including arrhythmia, angina, congestive heart failure and heart attacks. While there are other causes for these conditions, one common thread is atherosclerosis. In fact, atherosclerosis contributes to about three-quarters of all deaths related to heart disease. Here's an overview of how atherosclerosis develops, along with the other conditions it can lead to.

Atherosclerosis: Atherosclerosis is the build-up of plaque deposits inside the arteries. As you learned in Chapter 1, this plaque damages the arteries, causing them to become narrow and stiff. In the United States and most other Western countries, atherosclerosis is the leading cause of illness and death. In the United States alone, it caused almost 1 million deaths in 1992 – twice as many as from cancer and 10 times as many as from accidents.

Atherosclerosis begins when white blood cells called monocytes migrate from the bloodstream into the wall of the artery and are transformed into cells that accumulate fatty materials. In time, these fat-laden monocytes accumulate, leading to a patchy thickening of plaque in the inner lining of the artery. Each area of thickening is filled with a soft cheese-like substance consisting of cholesterol, smooth muscle cells and connective tissue cells. Plaque may be scattered throughout the medium and large arteries, but usually they form where the arteries branch off – presumably because the constant turbulence at these areas injures the arterial wall, making it more susceptible to plaque formation.

Arteries affected with atherosclerosis lose their elasticity, and as the plaques grow, the arteries narrow. Plaques can grow large enough to significantly reduce the blood's flow through an artery. But most of the damage occurs when they become fragile and rupture. Plaques that rupture cause blood clots to form that can block blood flow or break off and travel to another part of the body. If either happens and blocks a blood vessel that feeds the heart, it causes a heart attack. If it blocks a blood vessel that feeds the brain, it causes a stroke.

Arteriosclerosis: Often referred to as a "hardening of the arteries," arteriosclerosis actually defines several different, but related disorders. These disorders are marked by thickening of the arteries, loss of elasticity and hardening of the artery walls as calcium and plaque are deposited. As in atherosclerosis, these deposits narrow the arteries, thus interfering with the normal flow of blood through the vessel.

For years the cholesterol, fat and calcium deposited on the artery walls have been thought to be the mechanisms causing heart disease, and low-fat, low-cholesterol diets are commonly recommended. The end result of over ten years of these diet programs is an epidemic increase of fatter and sicker individuals. More logical and conclusive research recently shows that free radical damage to the artery walls initiates a natural repair sequence that results in the patching and buildup of calcium and cholesterol deposits.

Arteriosclerosis can happen to any artery, but is most serious in those vessels that channel blood to the heart and brain. When vessels to the heart narrow, not only is blood flow to the entire body diminished, but a lot of stress is placed on your heart to work harder as it tries to pump blood through the narrowing passages. Symptoms include leg cramps while walking, changes in skin temperature and color, an altered pulse, headaches, dizziness and memory defects. The problem is that symptoms often do not arise until the problem has progressed to a dangerous phase.

Angina Pectoris: Angina is a heavy, tight squeezing pain in the chest caused by insufficient oxygen supply to the heart (low blood flow to the heart). It generally occurs when the heart is working hard and requires more oxygen: during exercise, at times of stress, in extremes of temperature or soon after a meal. Typically the pain develops at the same point in daily activity; for example, while climbing stairs or at a certain point in your daily walk. The pain often radiates through the left shoulder, arm, or jaw and can last for up to 20 minutes. For some the pain might be intense, while others may feel only a mild discomfort. Some individuals have no symptoms at all. Irregardless of the level of discomfort, any angina is a gravely dangerous situation because it is often the precursor of a heart attack.

A TYPICAL ANGINA

Not all forms of angina have the same symptoms. Here are some not-so-typical signs to look for:

- Noctural angina (chest pain while resting)
- Prinzemetal angina (a coronary artery spasm)
- Pain in the jaw or ear
- Shortness of breath
- Indigestion

Cardiac Arrhythmia: Arrhythmias are abnormal or irregular heartbeats caused by a disturbance in the electrical nerve impulses of the heart. One cause of arrhythmia is arteriosclerosis, where deposits narrow the blood vessels and an inadequate blood supply reaches the heart. Valvular disease, high blood pressure, primary conduction abnormalities of the heart or myocardidis can all cause arrhythmia in the absence of atherosclerosis. Arrhythmias occur more frequently after a heart attack.

Congestive Heart Failure: Heart failure is a serious condition in which the heart is not pumping as well as it should. In other words, the heart is failing to pump efficiently and cannot meet the body's demand for oxygen, which often results in congestion in the lungs. When the heart can't pump enough oxygen-rich blood to function properly, it tries to overcompensate for the problem, which only makes things worse.

According to current statistics from the American Heart Association, there are five million heart failure patients in the United States, and 550,000 new cases of heart failure diagnosed in the United States every year. This includes 10 out every 1,000 people over the age of 65. Of all newly diagnosed patients, 50 percent of heart failure patients die within 5 years of diagnosis. Males and females appear to be affected about equally, but a disproportionate number of women die from the condition (62.3 percent of more than 45,000 deaths).

Heart Attack: Also known as myocardial infarction, a heart attack is the sudden death of part of the heart muscle. This is caused either by inflammation of the artery, hardening of the arteries or a sudden blood clot in an artery which leads to a deficiency of oxygen of the heart muscle and necrosis (muscle death).

Each year about 1 million people have a heart attack and one-third of those attacks are fatal. In developed countries, heart attacks are the single most common cause of death. Anyone who has suffered a heart attack has an increased risk of suffering another one in the following few years, especially if lifestyle and dietary changes are not made to reverse the factors that caused the first heart attack.

REMEMBER . . .

➤ Atherosclerosis (plaque buildup) contributes to three-quarters of all deaths related to heart disease.

➤ Arteries affected with atherosclerosis lose their elasticity and can become narrow enough to reduce blood flow.

➤ Plaques can rupture and cause blood clots which can lead to heart attack and stroke.

➤ Angina, or chest pain, is often felt in the left shoulder, arm or jaw and may signal an impending heart attack.

➤ An arrhythmia can be a symptom of atherosclerosis or high blood pressure and may occur more frequently after a heart attack.

➤ Congestive heart failure is a serious condition that occurs when the heart is not pumping as well as it should. Symptoms include shortness of breath and persistent coughing.

➤ Heart attacks are the leading cause of death and happen when part of the heart muscle dies suddenly. Signs of a heart attack include pressure in the chest, pain in one or both arms, back, neck, jaw or stomach, or shortness of breath, cold sweat, nausea and lightheadedness.

If you experience these symptoms, call 911 immediately.

Chapter 3
IN THE DOCTOR'S OFFICE

Go to any cardiologist and you'll likely be subjected to a battery of diagnostic tests. If the results show that you have a higher than average risk for heart disease, you'll probably leave the office with a fistful of prescriptions for statin drugs, ACE inhibitors, beta-blockers and blood thinners, along with some very conservative advice about diet and exercise (eat less dietary cholesterol and exercise more).

But, as is often the case, when these measures don't work, the doctor will probably order additional tests – more complex and more expensive. Often these tests convince your doctor that surgery or other invasive procedures, such as angioplasty or stent placement, is the only answer. So, depending on the test results, you schedule an angioplasty or maybe bypass surgery.

Although some heart problems can't be fixed by drugs or natural means, surgery should be the last resort. Unfortunately, that's often not the case, even though many cardiac surgeries are simply unnecessary and dangerous. And many of these operations don't prolong or improve the quality of a patient's life.

We've all heard of someone whose stent failed or who needs to have yet another risky bypass operation. While conventional medicine is learning that their methods aren't always the best medicine – as evidenced by the fact that bypass surgery rates dropped 50 percent in the early 1990s – they are learning far too slowly.

If you are at risk for heart disease, or have already been diagnosed with it, it's important to know the risks and benefits of the drugs or surgical procedures your doctor recommends. What you'll find below is an overview of the conventional options modern medicine has to offer:

Diagnostic Tests And Screening

➤ **Standard diagnostic testing**

- **Electrocardiogram (EKG):** Used to determine normal or abnormal heart rate and response.

- **Stress testing with EKG:** The well-known treadmill exercise test that helps determine the heart's reaction to an increased demand for oxygen.

- **Screening tests for heart disease and risk factors,** which include:

  - **Blood pressure**

  - **Cholesterol profile:** Measures total cholesterol, HDL (good) and LDL (bad) cholesterol, and triglycerides.

  - **HeartScoring:** Detects the presence of calcium buildup inside the major arteries of the heart.

➤ **Advanced diagnostic testing:**

- **Echocardiography:** Used to determine normal or abnormal blood flow through heart chambers and valves.

- **Stress echocardiogram:** Looks for evidence of previous heart muscle damage and finds any areas of the heart that have a decreased blood supply.

- **Stress testing with imaging:** Imaging, or nuclear scanning, of the heart shows how well blood flows to the heart muscle.

- **Holter monitoring:** A continuous EKG recording of heart rhythm during normal activity. This test may be done to determine how a patient is responding to cardiac medication.

- **Angiogram:** This special X-ray test is done to find the spot where a coronary artery is clogged. It can reveal how clogged the artery is and determine if the patient needs treatment such as angioplasty or coronary artery bypass surgery or drug therapy.

The Pros & Cons of Prescription Drugs

Drugs are one of the cornerstones of conventional medicine, especially when it comes to heart disease. While prescription drugs can be lifesaving under some circumstances, too often doctors hand them out like candy – commonly in place of, or in conjunction with, the recommendation to change your diet or exercise habits.

Don't get me wrong. I'm not opposed to the use of drugs to treat heart disease. But, in their blind acceptance of the benefits drugs provide, modern medicine relies far too heavily on them. If they are so effective, why are high blood pressure and unhealthy cholesterol levels rampant? And why are heart attacks still the No. 1 cause of death in the U.S.?

Not only are drugs *not* the magic bullet many folks in the mainstream medical community believe they are, many of them only treat the symptoms of heart disease instead of the root cause. Of more concern, prescription drugs carry a host of adverse side effects. Let's take a look at the benefits and drawbacks of the main types of drugs commonly used to treat heart disease.

ACE Inhibitors: Technically known as angiotensin-converting enzyme inhibitors, these drugs are often prescribed to relieve the symptoms of congestive heart failure or to lower blood pressure. People who have suffered from a heart attack may also receive ACE inhibitors since some studies

Side Effects of ACE Inhibitors

- Dry cough
- Large drop in blood pressure
- Kidney and liver problems
- Rash
- Inflammation of the pancreas
- Sinusitis
- Sore throat
- Gastrointestinal upset
- Changes in blood cells

have shown that they may prevent further damage to the heart muscle.

These drugs work by blocking angiotensin II. Angiotensin II is the chemical responsible for narrowing blood vessels and raising blood pressure. The body produces angiotensin II by converting another chemical called angiotensin I. It is the angiotensin-converting enzyme (ACE) that makes this reaction possible. By blocking - or inhibiting - the action of that enzyme, the conversion to angiotensin II is interrupted and blood pressure is lowered.

Older people may show an exaggerated drop in blood pressure after the first dose of an ACE inhibitor. Therefore, many doctors give patients a short-acting ACE inhibitor such as Captropril and watch their blood pressure for several hours. Longer-acting ACE inhibitors are given when the patient's tolerance to Captropril is established.

ACE inhibitors can cause serum potassium levels to rise, so patients on this type of medication should avoid taking supplemental potassium. And if you are taking an arthritis drug, be aware that some can make ACE inhibitors less effective.

Beta-Blockers: Beta-adrenergic blockers or "beta blockers" are a family of drugs used to treat high blood pressure, angina and heart arrhythmia. Beta-blockers "block" the effects of adrenaline on your body's beta receptors. This slows the nerve impulses that travel through the

Side Effects of Beta-Blockers

- Drowsiness
- Dizziness
- Cold hands and feet
- Dry mouth
- Shortness of breath
- Insomnia
- Digestive problems
- Depression
- Memory loss
- Erectile dysfunction

heart. As a result, your heart does not have to work as hard because it needs less blood and oxygen. Beta-blockers also block the impulses that can cause an arrhythmia.

People with asthma, chronic bronchitis, emphysema or other respiratory conditions should avoid beta-blockers since they can make these conditions worse by narrowing the air passages in the lungs. In people with already reduced heart function, beta blockers may decrease the pumping ability of their heart enough to cause heart failure.

Beta-blockers interact with a number of other medications, including anaesthetics and non-steroidal anti-inflammatory drugs (NSAIDS). Taking antiarrhythmics can increase the heart slowing effects of beta-blockers. And certain cough and cold remedies and appetite suppressants can cause a dramatic rise in blood pressure if taken with a beta-blocker.

Blood Thinners: Despite their name, these drugs do not thin the blood. They do however, prevent the blood from clotting – hence they are known as anticoagulants. Aspirin is probably the best known and most widely used blood thinner.

The September 22, 2003 issue of the journal *Archives of Internal Medicine* published the results of a meta-analysis of five major clinical trials which confirmed that aspirin plays an important role in heart attack prevention. Since that time three more trials

Side Effects of Blood Thinners

- Stomach upset
- Peptic ulcer
- Tendency to bruise
- Allergic reactions
- Bleeding
- Abdominal pain
- Upper respiratory infection
- Depression
- High cholesterol
- Irregular heartbeat
- Hepatitis

concerning aspirin's primary prevention benefits have been published. One of the studies analyzed data from 55,580 randomized participants and found a 32 percent reduction in heart attack and a 15 percent combined reduction in the risk of heart attack, stroke and vascular death associated with aspirin use.

But British researchers at the Wolfson Institute of Preventive Medicine aren't nearly as gung-ho on recommending aspirin to everyone at risk for a heart attack, especially if they have high blood pressure. Their study included 5,000 men, age 45 to 69 years, who were at risk of coronary heart disease but had not previously had heart trouble. The men were randomly divided into four different treatment groups to accurately establish the effect of aspirin.

The Wolfson team found that those men with low blood pressure got more benefit from taking aspirin than those with high blood pressures, not only for coronary heart disease but also for stroke. They also noted that men with higher pressures may derive no protective benefit from aspirin. And, according to the Wolfson researchers, even a modest benefit provided by aspirin doesn't necessarily outweigh the risk of bleeding.

Although most of us consider aspirin safe, it isn't without risk. According to new evidence, many people who take aspirin for a heart condition appear to have an unexpectedly high risk of serious cardiac problems when they stop the medication, even on a doctor's order. A recent French study included a review of 1,236 people hospitalized for heart attacks and other acute coronary events. Of that group, 500 of them had been taking aspirin on their doctor's orders. In that subgroup, 51, or slightly more than 10 percent, were hospitalized within a week after they stopped taking the drug. Twenty of those patients had stopped taking the aspirin without consulting their physicians. But the others were obeying doctors' orders to avoid potential bleeding problems during such medical procedures as dental work or minor surgery.

If aspirin doesn't sufficiently prevent blood clots or if you've already suffered from a heart attack, your doctor may prescribe either Coumadin (warfarin) or Plavix (clopidogrel bisulfate). Both of these pharmaceuticals prevent clotting, but there are some important differences.

Plavix interferes with the normal functioning platelets so they resist clumping together or sticking to damaged, irregular areas within the blood vessel wall. Plavix is used following specific cardiovascular procedures such as stent supported angioplasty or for patients who have had a recent stroke or heart attack. But because this drug slows clotting, it can take longer than usual to stop bleeding.

Coumadin, on the other hand, interferes with the purely chemical reaction that causes blood to thicken at an injury site. It is commonly given to patients who have mechanical heart valves, stents in the pulmonary artery or chronic atrial flutter. But Coumadin may increase the risk of plaque breaking away from artery walls and lodging at another point, causing a blockage. Coumadin also interacts with a wide variety of drugs, supplements and herbs, including vitamin C, magnesium, garlic and ginkgo biloba.

Calcium Channel Blockers: These drugs are usually

Side Effects of Calcium Channel Blockers

- Headache
- Flushing
- Constipation
- Nausea
- Potassium loss
- High cholesterol
- Swelling in the lower extremities
- Low blood pressure
- Liver problems
- Heart attack
- Cancer

prescribed to treat high blood pressure, angina and arrhythmia. They work by slowing down the rate that calcium enters the heart and vessel walls. As a result, the arteries relax and dilate, allowing the blood to flow more easily. This lowers the demands on the heart and improves circulation, which in turn lowers blood pressure.

While calcium channel blockers come with a host of side effects, these problems are minor compared to those found in a 1995 study by the University of Wisconsin. In the study, 623 hypertensive patients who had experienced a heart attack were compared with 2,032 patients with high blood pressure but no heart attack. They found that those patients taking a calcium channel blocker had a 60 percent higher incidence in heart attacks than those taking other hypertension drugs.

If that weren't bad enough, a recent review of nine calcium channel blocker trials found that patients taking these drugs had a significantly higher risk of heart attack, congestive heart failure and other cardiovascular events. The study's authors concluded that "calcium antagonists are inferior to other types of antihypertensive drugs as first-line agents in reducing the risks of several major complications of hypertension and should not be recommended as first-line therapy for hypertension." Yet these are often the first choice of doctors for the treatment of high blood pressure.

Long-term and seemingly unrelated risks have also been linked to the use of calcium channel blockers. According to a study by Catholic University in Rome, the long-term use of calcium channel blockers is linked to the development of cancer, especially lung, colon, urinary tract, prostate and breast cancer. And a new study of post-menopausal women taking calcium channel blockers by the Fred Hutchinson Cancer Research Center in Seattle found that these medications double the risk of breast cancer in older women – and if a woman was also on estrogen, the risk jumped to more than eight times that of women not taking calcium channel blockers.

Cholesterol Lowering Drugs: Cholesterol-lowering drugs are used to treat people with higher-than-normal levels of cholesterol in their blood when dietary restrictions, lifestyle changes and weight reduction don't do the trick. These drugs, known as statins, work by blocking an enzyme called HMG-CoA reductase, which causes the body to make LDL cholesterol.

But statin drugs also have a dark side. It seems that the same enzymes involved in the production of cholesterol are also required for the production of coenzyme Q10. Not surprisingly, lower cholesterol levels in statin users are accompanied by a depletion of CoQ10. CoQ10 plays an important role in providing energy to the cells, especially in the heart – and low levels are implicated in virtually all cardiovascular diseases, including angina, hypertension, cardiomyopathy and congestive heart failure.

HEART SMART TIP

THE STATIN SCAM

Many of my colleagues insist that statins can lower CRP. They cite a single study conducted at Walter Reed Army Medical Center. Of 130 heart-attack victims in the study, those who received a statin drug had significantly lower CRP levels – up to 36 percent lower.

But this one study isn't nearly enough evidence to explain the dozens of patients who walk into my office with high CRP levels *after their doctor put them on statins*!

What statins can do is increase the risk of cataracts and weaken your immune system. Take my advice – avoid statin drugs at all costs.

If you have high cholesterol, check Chapter 8 for safe and natural ways to reign in your levels.

Statin drugs can also cause rhabdomyolysis, a life-threatening condition that destroys muscle cells and releases them into the bloodstream, a condition that can eventually cause fatal kidney failure. Rhabdomyolysis gained national attention when it was linked to Baycol, the statin drug that was pulled from the market in 2001 after causing more then 100 deaths and 1,600 injuries.

Rhabdomyolysis isn't the only condition triggered by statins. Researchers at the University of Pittsburgh have reported that lova-statin could affect attention and reaction speed. In their study, patients whose cholesterol had been lowered with lovastatin paid less attention and had delayed psychomotor reflexes compared with those who had not received the drug. Those who had the greatest decreases in cholesterol levels suffered the greatest impairment.

Statins have also been found to suppress certain immune system cells known as helper T-cells. Helper T-cells act by recognizing foreign pathogens and then activating the production of the proper immune cells in response. And a recent multinational study has found that statin drugs increase the risk of cataracts, especially in patients who are also taking antibiotics.

Side Effects of Cholesterol Lowering Drugs

- Headache
- Insomnia
- Liver problems
- Abdominal pain
- Nausea
- Diarrhea
- Gas
- Skin rash
- Immune problems
- Hepatitis
- Rhabdomyolysis

Despite mounting evidence that these drugs are unsafe, there are 13 million Americans using statins, making it the most widely prescribed class of anti-cholesterol drugs on the market.

Digitalis: This natural derivative from the foxglove plant is used to treat congestive heart failure and arrhythmias. Digitalis can increase blood flow throughout your body and reduce swelling in your hands and ankles.

Digitalis works in two ways. First it strengthens the force of

Side Effects of Digitalis
• Dizziness
• Shortness of breath
• Heart palpitations
• Sweating
• Fainting
• Hallucinations
• Confusion
• Depression
• Visual changes
• Breast enlargement in men
• Erectile dysfunction

the heartbeat by increasing the amount of calcium in the heart's cells. When the medicine reaches the heart muscle, it binds to sodium and potassium receptors. These receptors control the amount of calcium in the heart muscle by stopping the mineral from leaving the cells. As calcium builds up in the cells, it causes a stronger heartbeat. Digitalis also helps control irregular heart rhythms by slowing the electrical signals that travel through the heart and regulates the number of heartbeats.

Although this drug originally comes from a natural herb (foxglove), the modern form of digitalis is anything but natural. It is a synthetic medication known as digoxin and sold under the name lanoxin.

It has been reported that, when digoxin is combined with certain anti-arrhythmic drugs, and calcium channel blockers sudden death can occur. While digitalis can interact with other medications, you should also avoid caffeine, diet pills, laxatives and cough, cold, and sinus medicines.

Nitrates: These drugs are used to prevent and temporarily relieve angina by expanding the arteries. They may also be used to lower blood pressure and improve heart function. Millions of Americans with

Side Effects of Nitrates

- Flushing
- Headache
- Restlessness
- Insomnia
- Nightmares
- Heart attack

coronary artery disease have been prescribed nitrate-based drugs. The best known, of course, is nitroglycerin. But there are nearly 30 other nitrate drugs that doctors can choose from. Available in tablet, capsule, patch or ointment form, the difference in these drugs is how quickly they work to ease chest pain.

While there's no doubt that these drugs work, new evidence suggests that the regular use of nitrate drugs actually increase the risk of future heart attack. This startling new finding came from a Japanese study that involved 518 patients with suspected coronary artery disease. The patients were divided into groups based on the degree of arterial damage (endothelial dysfunction) and how often they used nitrate drugs. After tracking the patients for 45 months, the researchers discovered something unexpected – those who regularly used nitrate drugs were 2.42 times more likely to suffer major cardiovascular events. The doctors concluded that the effects of nitrate drugs accelerate atherogenic processes and endothelial dysfunction and that nitrate drug use causes future cardiovascular events.

Of course, this study referred to the use of nitrates on a regular basis, not the occasional use of these drugs. But even occasional use can lead to problems. Combining nitroglycerin with impotence drugs like Viagra and Levitra can result in dangerously low blood pressure and has been linked to heart attacks and more than 500 deaths.

Vasodilators: Like nitrates, vasodilators act directly on the muscles in blood vessel walls to make blood vessels widen. By widening the arteries, these drugs allow blood to flow through more easily, reducing blood pressure.

Vasodilators, like hydralazine (Apresoline) and minoxidil (Loniten), aren't a permanent fix for high blood pressure, but they can help control the condition. Unfortunately, they may also worsen the problems that result from heart disease, blood vessel disease, or a recent heart attack or stroke. This medicine may also make angina worse.

Side Effects of Vasodilators
• Headaches
• Nausea or vomiting
• Loss of appetite
• Bloating
• Joint and muscle pain
• Swollen lymph nodes
• Fever
• Chest pain
• Possible birth defects

Is Surgery The Answer?

Sometime drugs aren't enough to tame heart disease. And that's when, according to conventional medicine, it's time for surgery. But like drugs, surgery only addresses the symptoms of heart disease, not the root cause. Worse yet, coronary bypass and cardiovascular procedures, including balloon angioplasty and stent implantation are risky and often unnecessary.

Here's a classic example: B. G., a friend of mine and someone with whom I competed with in many triathlons in the early 1980s, recently suffered from severe chest pain after his morning workout. After being admitted to the hospital, tests discovered the cause of B.G.'s heart attack – a clot in one of the branches of his left anterior descending coronary artery. The cardiologist cleaned out the clot, inserted a stent to open up the artery and sent him home two days later. Two weeks later, B.G. called me and said, "Bob, I'm having chest pains again!" I told him to call 911 and get to the hospital immediately. I knew he was having another heart attack. Why was he having this second heart attack? According to his doctor, he had clotted his stent!

> # WHAT'S IN A NAME?
>
> Most patients are under the mistaken impression that all cardiac procedures are done by a cardiac surgeon. Nothing could be further from the truth!
>
> Cardiac surgeons *only* perform cardiac bypass surgery or open heart surgery. Angioplasty, atherectomies and stent placements are all done by a cardiologist.

We all know of someone who has had a bypass or angioplasty – they've become common terms in modern lexicon. But most of us don't really know the whys and wherefores of cardiac surgery. So let's look at the most common surgical "fixes" used today.

Atherectomy: Used to remove plaque, atherectomies are sometimes thought of as the Roto-Rooter of cardiac medicine. During the procedure, the cardiologist places a catheter into the artery which is equipped with one of several tools to clean out the damaging plaque. This type of surgery is usually performed when plaque has become very hard.

Once the catheter is in place, the cardiologist cuts away the plaque using a either a sharp blade or abrasive material (like sandpaper) located at the tip of the catheter. As the plaque is removed, the bits and pieces are stored in a tiny container which is removed when the catheter is withdrawn from the artery. This technique is useful in larger arteries with "softer" plaque.

Another tool used in atherectomies is a rotoblator, which quickly grinds the plaque into very small particles. In most cases, these microparticles can travel safely through the circulatory system. But if a clot is present, your cardiologist may opt for a transluminal extraction catheter, which sucks the plaque particles into a vacuum and expels them from the body. No matter what method the cardiologist uses, many atherectomies are followed by balloon angioplasty and stenting.

By removing some of the plaque, blood flow is improved, which can relieve angina and even help prevent heart attacks and death. However, without lifestyle changes, it's likely plaque will reform over time.

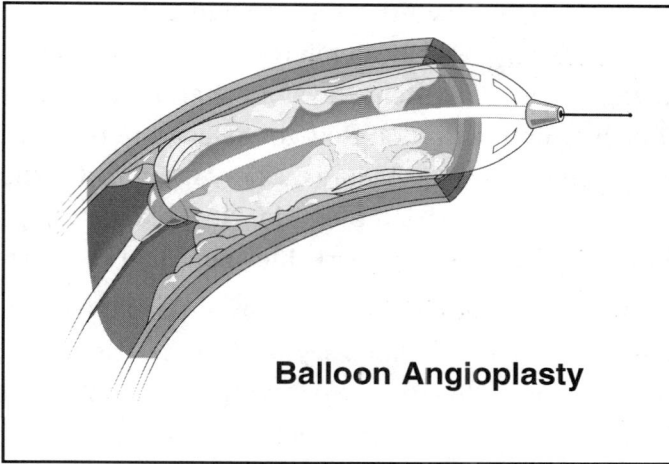

Balloon Angioplasty

The chance of serious complications during an atherectomy is quite small, but this type of procedure is riskier than other catheter-based surgeries like balloon angioplasties. Serious complications can include abrupt vessel closure, the need for emergency bypass surgery or a heart attack. Atherectomies may also result in a perforation of a blood vessel or can cause a blockage created by loose particles of plaque.

Angioplasty: Balloon angioplasty is a well-established procedure that can be effective for some patients. In fact, it's become so routine that its use has tripled since 1987.

This type of procedure is used to dilate narrowed arteries. A doctor inserts and advances a catheter with a deflated balloon at its tip into the narrowed part of an artery. Then the balloon is inflated, compressing the plaque and enlarging the inner diameter of the blood vessel so blood can flow more easily.

Numerous studies show that angioplasties can improve angina and exercise tolerance in heart patients. However, research shows that this type of surgery can also increase the risk of more serious cardiac events and death.

In 1999, one million balloon angioplasties were performed in the U.S. Of those, at least 70 percent included placing a stent in the artery. Stents are wire mesh tubes used to prop open arteries after an angioplasty. The stent stays in the artery permanently, holds it open, improves blood flow to the heart muscle and relieves symptoms. The problem is, as my friend B.G. knows all too well, stents can fail – and often do. New plaque can grow around the wire mesh with remarkable speed and clog the artery.

Even with stenting, about 40 percent of people who've had an angioplasty find that the dilated segment of the artery narrows again (a condition called restenosis) within six months after the procedure. And, in many cases, there are no symptoms. According to a study at Green Lane Hospital in Auckland, New Zealand, more than half of all patients whose arteries re-narrow have no symptoms and, as a consequence, have a silent risk of a future heart attack. Although another angioplasty might fix the problem if it is identified, most doctors recommend coronary artery bypass surgery.

Another problem with stents is the metal with which they are made. A study conducted at University Hospital Eppendorf in Hamburg, Germany has found that stainless steel coronary stents may trigger allergic reactions to substances such as nickel, molybdenum or chromium. Of the 89 patients who experienced restenosis, 10 had an allergic reaction to either molybdenum or nickel. These findings led the researchers to conclude that allergic reactions may be a major factor in causing in-stent restenosis.

While angioplasty and stenting might sound good on paper, when it comes to their safety and efficacy in people, this medical experiment has been a huge failure. At the American Heart Association meeting on interventional cardiology in 1998, Dr. James E Tcheng, Associate Professor at Duke University Medical Center, said, "For those of you who think that stent implantation is the 'end all and be all,' because it creates a perfect environment that cannot support a thrombus, I would suggest that assumption is wrong. What we are doing [with intervention] is creating heart attacks. Whenever you are blowing up a balloon in a patient's artery, activating a rotablator or turning on a laser, you are causing damage to the inside of the vessel. This sets your patient up for platelet adhesion and aggregation, vasoactive substance release, thrombus formation and the potential for abrupt closure and development of acute ischemic syndrome."

SAFETY ALERT!

Despite serious problems, coating stents with drugs is all the rage among cardiologists. As a result many doctors are experimenting with this experimental device, using the new stents aggressively and inappropriately. In some cases, they either use the wrong size stent for the size of the artery or place a stent in patients who don't need it.

The new drug-coated stents may not be any better. In the rush to build a better mousetrap, the FDA approved these devices after a study found that stents coated with the drug paclitaxel reduced return arterial narrowing better than stents without the drug. But that study was small, only 176 patients, and a larger trial failed to confirm the effect. Nevertheless, over 50,000 drug-coated stents have been used in patients during the first three months following its approval. But, even though these devices appear to reduce restenosis, some scientists are concerned that drug-coated stents may not be preventing restenosis, but only delaying it. Another, more serious problem is that these stents can clot within days of being implanted. On October 28, 2003, the Food and Drug Administration (FDA) issued a warning letter to physicians about blood clots and other side effects associated with drug-coated stents, noting that these devices were responsible for more than 360 cases of thrombosis (blood clots). Of those, more than 70 patients died.

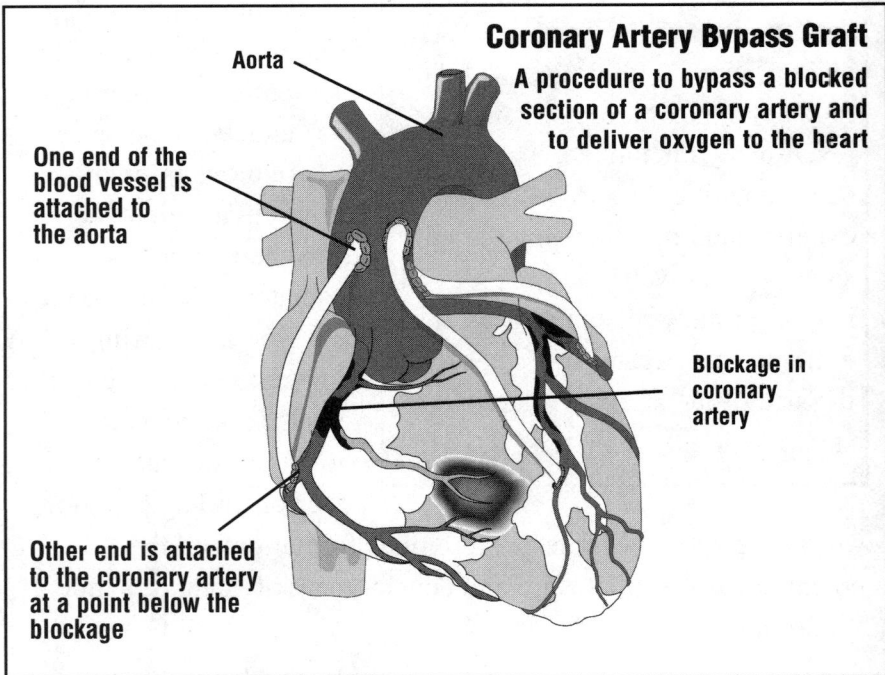

Coronary Artery Bypass Graft

A procedure to bypass a blocked section of a coronary artery and to deliver oxygen to the heart

Aorta

One end of the blood vessel is attached to the aorta

Blockage in coronary artery

Other end is attached to the coronary artery at a point below the blockage

In other cases, the stent was associated with injuries requiring medical or surgical intervention. The FDA has received more than 50 reports (some relating to deaths) concerning allergic or hypersensitive reactions to drug-coated stents. The symptoms include pain, rash, respiratory problems, hives, itching, fever and blood pressure changes.

As far as I'm concerned, both the bare wire and drug-coated stents are still experimental, despite their widespread use. Instead of becoming a guinea pig, the best thing to do is to avoid stents in the first place by following the recommendations in this book.

Coronary Artery Bypass: This surgery reroutes, or "bypasses," blood around clogged arteries to improve blood flow and oxygen to the heart. The surgeon takes a segment of healthy blood vessel from another part of the body (typically the leg) and makes a detour around the blocked part of the coronary artery.

Depending on which blood vessel is used, one end is either sewn to the aorta or remains connected to the larger artery it originated from. The other end is attached (grafted) beyond the blockage in the artery. As a result, blood can flow around the blocked area, increasing the supply of oxygen and nutrients to the heart muscle.

For patients with severe angina who are unable to participate in normal activities or someone who doesn't respond to medication, a coronary bypass may be the only option. However, people who suffer from stable angina or those who find relief through medication should opt for a second opinion since neither of these scenarios are an indication for surgery.

> ## HEART SMART TIP
>
> Research shows that total blockage is 16 times more common in arteries after bypass surgery then in those that have been left alone. That's why I always advocate getting a second – or even a third – opinion before agreeing to undergo this risky surgery.

Short-term complications can include difficulty breathing, bleeding, infection, high blood pressure and abnormal heart rhythm. More serious complications that may arise include heart attack, stroke or even death. These risks are higher for older patients, diabetics, patients with other major health problems and those undergoing a repeat bypass procedure.

While it's true that bypass surgery can ease pain, the relief is often temporary. Since bypass surgery doesn't actually slow atherosclerosis, the disease progresses and the pain inevitably returns. While three-quarters of bypass patients remain pain-free for three to nine months after the procedure, according to an investigation by George Washington University, 45 percent of the patients studied experienced mild symptoms and 32 percent suffered from severe pain within five years of this surgery. Worse yet, atherosclerosis speeds up in arteries that have received grafts. In one study, arteries with grafts develop a complete blockage in 40 percent of cases compared to only 6 percent in people without grafts.

Another serious problem many bypass patients experience is cognitive impairment, including difficulty following directions, memory problems, personality changes, mood swings and irritability. Researchers at Duke University confirm that persistent mental changes are quite common after bypass surgery. They found that six months after surgery, 25 percent of the patients still showed signs of decreased mental function.

Side Effects of Pacemakers

- Dizziness
- Fatigue
- Bacterial infection
- Bleeding
- Blood clot
- Tearing of a blood vessel
- Stroke
- Heart attack
- Malfunction

Defibrillators: Most of us are familiar with the defibrillators used in hospitals to "jumpstart" the heart of a patient in cardiac arrest. In fact, medical TV shows make great hay out of whipping out the paddles and shocking a patient back to life.

But, for patients suffering from chronic arrhythmias involving ventricular tachycardia or ventricular fibrillation, there is a type of defibrillator that can be surgically implanted in a patient's chest. This tiny implantable cardioverter defibrillator (ICD) monitors the heart and, if necessary, corrects an abnormally fast or "quivering" heartbeat at the first sign of a problem.

Although inserting a defibrillator is considered minor surgery, it can result in the formation of a blood clot, a torn blood vessel, heart attack or stroke. These risks are greater in older people or in those who are obese.

Pacemakers: Even though the heart has its own natural pacemaker that sets its rhythm, the term "pacemaker" most commonly refers to an artificial electronic device that is implanted in the chest to regulate the heart's rhythm. Generally, pacemakers correct an abnormally slow heartbeat by sending electrical impulses to one or more chambers of the heart. These signals make the heart contract at a more regular rhythm than the chamber would otherwise.

Nearly 200,000 pacemakers are implanted annually in the United States. In most cases, people with pacemakers enjoy a significant improvement in their quality of life. But there are some environments they must avoid, including metal detectors, MRI machines and slot machines. Cell phones should be held at least 6 inches from the pacemaker at all times, even if the phone is turned off.

Some people face the risk of developing "pacemaker syndrome," in which the implanted pacemaker is no longer synchronized with the heart's own rhythm and attempts to pump blood through a closed valve. This restricts the flow of blood from the heart, causing dizziness and fatigue in the patient. It occurs in one of four users of the *single chamber* pacemaker (one that stimulates one chamber of the heart), but there is no risk of this syndrome for users of the *double-chamber* pacemaker (which stimulates two chambers of the heart).

A recent study suggests that up to 20 percent of patients with pacemakers or other implanted devices are at a high risk of developing bacterial blood infections. Sometimes the device itself is the cause of the infection. The FDA has issued a number of advisories on the incidence of staph infection within six years of a pacemaker being inserted. Another cause for concern is that recalls for pacemakers increased over the past decade. The FDA has issued safety alerts affecting 400,000 pacemakers and more than 100,000 ICDs.

Although these procedures are sometimes necessary, you may be able to avoid them by preventing heart disease in the first place. The key is to adopt the strategies found in the following chapters: eat a healthy diet, exercise, lower stress and take heart-friendly supplements.

What if you already suffer from some form of heart disease? While cardiac surgery has its place in medicine, if your doctor recommends any of the above procedures, get a second opinion. If the surgery's benefits outweigh the risks, then, and only then, should it be considered.

REMEMBER . . .

➤ Drugs are not a magic bullet and most carry a host of side effects.

➤ Although many people rely on aspirin to prevent heart attacks, this over-the-counter drug isn't harmless. Long-term use has been linked to excessive bleeding and ulcers.

➤ If possible, avoid taking statin drugs to lower cholesterol. But if you must, make sure you take supplemental Co-Q10 since statins can deplete this important nutrient.

➤ Some cardiovascular drugs, especially calcium channel blockers and nitrates, can actually increase the risk of heart attack.

➤ Many heart medications can adversely interact with other drugs, foods or supplements.

➤ Be aware of all your options before agreeing to invasive cardiac procedures or bypass surgery.

➤ Stents often fail and may be dangerous. The new drug-coated stents may also cause blood clots.

➤ Bypass surgery may only offer temporary relief from chest pain and can accelerate atherosclerosis.

➤ Total arterial blockage is 16 times more common *after* bypass surgery.

➤ The bottom line: Avoid invasive procedures unless at least two, possibly even three, cardiologists recommend the procedure.

Chapter 4
HEART HEALTHY EATING

The old adage that "you are what you eat" is especially true when it comes to your heart. Adopting a heart-healthy diet is one of the most important steps you can take to prevent heart disease.

Unlike drugs, which only treat the symptoms of heart disease, eating the right foods will provide your body with the nutrients it needs to prevent, even reverse, the risk factors for heart disease. You'll also see an increase in overall health and vitality. But, before we look at the way food impacts our health, let's address a problem that has become a health epidemic.

The Obesity Factor

In a nation obsessed with dieting, you might think we would all be thin, fit and healthy. But the truth is, more than three in five Americans are overweight, and nearly one in three is obese. It's no wonder high blood pressure, unhealthy cholesterol levels and heart disease are at all time highs.

Excess weight lowers the age of first heart attack. A 10-year study at the Mayo Clinic shows that merely being overweight drops the age of first heart attack by more than three and a half years. And if you're obese, you can expect to suffer a heart attack 8.2 years earlier than someone at normal weight.

Along with putting a strain on the heart, weight gain – particularly in the abdominal area – raises CRP levels. But, as University of Vermont investigators discovered, dropping excess pounds can also drop CRP. During their 14-month study, the scientists measured the CRP levels in 61 middle-aged women before putting them on a weight-loss program. In the women who lost an average of 33 pounds, CRP levels dropped by an astounding 32 percent. The more weight the women lost, the more their CRP levels fell.

When it comes to losing weight, a little can mean a lot. A modest weight loss of five to 10 percent of body weight can lower blood pressure and provide other health benefits even to the very obese, say scientists at the University Hospital of Antwerp in Belgium, who looked at several studies measuring the effect of modest weight loss on blood pressure. For a 250 pound man, that means just 25 pounds.

If you want to win at losing weight, forget fad diets or starvation schemes. Instead, set a goal of losing one to two pounds a week. Most women can achieve this by consuming 1,200 to 1,500 calories a day. Most men can lose the same amount by consuming 1,500 to 1,800 calories a day.

But that may be easier said than done. The typical American diet seems to undermine our efforts at every turn. Filled with salt, fat, refined grains and sugar, it's a prescription for disaster. In the following sections, I'm going to tell you about two of the worst dietary offenders for the health of your heart – salt and fat.

Shaking Out The Truth

Salt junkies are quick to point out that this tasty mineral is necessary for life. They're right, of course. Salt is naturally present in every cell in our bodies, in the fluid that surrounds cells and also in our bones. Sodium aids in muscle contraction and nerve transmission, helps transport carbon dioxide and moves amino acids from the gut to cells throughout the body.

HEART SMART TIP

What the Labels Mean

An easy way to reduce the amount of salt in your diet is to learn what the terms really mean:

Sodium-Free	5 mg. or less
Very-Low Sodium	35 mg. or less
Low Sodium	140 mg. or less
Reduced Sodium	25% less sodium
Light Sodium	50% less sodium

But, the problem with this line of thinking is that, when it comes to salt, a little goes a very long way. In fact, we only need 1,000 to 2,000 mg. of salt a day – much lower than the typical 7,000 to 15,000 mg. of salt most of us consume.

Preliminary evidence has linked high salt consumption with an increased incidence of cardiovascular disease and death among overweight people. In fact, a daily increase of just 2,300 mg. of excess sodium (bear in mind that a single teaspoon of salt contains 1,938 mg. of sodium) can increase your risk of dying from heart disease by a whopping 40 to 60 percent! Why? Because too much salt can dramatically raise your blood pressure.

An interesting study conducted by the National Heart, Lung, and Blood Institute recently found that those people who ate less salt significantly reduced their blood pressure, regardless of where blood pressure levels were when they began. In fact, the people who consumed 1,500 mg. a day or less showed the biggest drop, and thus greatly lessened their chances of ever developing high blood pressure.

So, we can all be healthier if we just leave the salt shaker in the cupboard, right? If only it were that easy. Nutritional experts say that only 10 percent of dietary sodium comes from adding salt to food at the dinner table. Instead, the bulk of sodium in our diet comes from prepared, processed and pickled foods. Lunch meats, prepared cheese, soda pop, canned soups and vegetables, condiments, salad dressings and baked goods can all be deceptively high in sodium.

Along with reducing the amount of salt you consume, you can minimize the negative impact of too much sodium by eating more potassium. Foods that are particularly high in potassium include fruits (apricots, avocado, bananas, dates, melons, oranges and peaches), vegetables (artichokes, broccoli, brussels sprouts, potatoes, pumpkin, spinach, sweet potatoes and winter squash) dried beans, peas and lentils.

The Skinny On Fats

Ask anyone what the most hated nutrient in America is and they'll probably say fat. For the last 20 years, fat has been linked to obesity, heart disease, colon cancer and diabetes. The problem is that fat also performs some critical functions in the body. It cushions and protects our vital organs and serves as building blocks for cell membranes. Certain essential fatty acids are indispensable to the prostaglandins and hormones that regulate numerous body functions. They are also required for the absorption of the fat-soluble vitamins A, D, E and K. But not all fats are created equal. To help sort out which kinds of fat we need and which ones contribute to disease, let's look at the different types of fat.

Saturated fat is primarily found in animal and dairy products (although some vegetable products like coconut oil, palm oil and vegetable shorting are also high in saturated fat). The liver uses saturated fat to make cholesterol, so consuming excessive amounts of foods high in saturated fats can significantly raise blood cholesterol levels, especially LDL, the "bad" cholesterol. You can always tell if a fat is saturated because it solidifies at room temperature.

Polyunsaturated fats are found in corn, soybean, safflower and sunflower oils. Some fish oils are also high in polyunsaturates. Unlike saturated fats, polyunsaturates may actually lower your total blood cholesterol level. The trouble is, they can also lower HDL (good) cholesterol levels. But polyunsaturated fats play a special role in human health because they supply essential fatty acids (EFAs). As their name implies, EFAs are indispensable to body function and must be supplied by the diet because our bodies can't manufacture them.

There are two major deficiencies of EFAs: omega-6 linoleic acid and omega-3 alpha-linolenic acid. Although most experts

HEART SMART TIP

Stock Up On EFAs

Essential fatty acids – specifically omega-6 and omega-3 EFAs, are key players in the conversion of food to energy, the transfer of oxygen to cells, the formation and maintenance of cell membranes, and the production of hormone-like prostaglandins, which guard against conditions such as cancer and heart disease. As a bonus, adequate EFA intake will help guard against depression, reduce inflammation, and give you healthy nails, hair and skin, faster healing and a more efficient level of fat burning.

The optimum daily dose is only 9 to 18 grams of omega-6 and 2 to 9 grams of omega-3, which can take the form of a single tablespoon of flaxseed or hemp oil in oatmeal in the morning, or a splash of walnut-oil vinaigrette on a lunchtime salad.

- Select organic and unrefined essential fatty acids
- Only buy oils that are packaged in protective opaque containers
- Store EFAs in the refrigerator
- Shoot for a daily intake of 2 to 9 grams of omega-3 and 9 to 18 grams of omega-6
- Discard oils if they start to change color or smell rancid
- Do not cook with oils—high heat destroys EFAs.

agree that omega-6 and omega-3 EFAs should be consumed in a 4:1 ratio, most people overdo omega-6 EFAs and consume far too few omega-3s. Omega-6 EFAs are found in most nuts (except peanuts) and seeds, and in vegetable oils such as sunflower and safflower oils. Sources of omega-3 fatty acids include flaxseeds and flaxseed oil, pumpkin seeds, walnuts and cold-water fish. To get both omega-6 and omega-3 fatty acids from one source, try hemp oil. Hemp provides a 3:1 ratio of omega-6 to omega-3 and has a wonderful nutty flavor that's great in salad dressings.

Monounsaturated fats are found mostly in vegetable and nut oils like olive, peanut and canola. These fats appear to reduce blood levels of LDLs without affecting HDLs in any way. But they don't lower LDL significantly, so monounsaturated fats should still be used sparingly.

While the body only requires small amounts of these fats to keep it humming along, there is one type of fat the body doesn't need at all. *Trans fatty acids*, or trans fats, are shaped differently than the polyunsaturated fatty acids from which they are made, and they adversely affect cell membranes and prostaglandin functions. In other words, trans fats act exactly the same as saturated fats in your body.

Numerous studies have found that trans-fatty acids raise total cholesterol, lower "good" HDL cholesterol, increase "bad" LDL cholesterol, interfere with blood sugar and insulin, and decrease immune function. Researchers at the University of Washington now report that high levels of trans-fatty acids are strongly associated with an increased risk of sudden cardiac death.

Their study involved 179 sudden cardiac death victims between the ages of 25 and 74 and 285 age- and sex-matched controls. Both cases and controls had blood samples drawn and analyzed for fatty acid levels in red blood cell membranes. The researchers found that cardiac arrest victims tended to have significantly higher overall levels of trans-fatty acids than did the controls. Specifically, they had higher levels of oleic and linoleic trans-fatty acids and significantly lower levels of beneficial omega-3 fatty acids. After adjusting for EFAs and other factors which could affect heart disease, they concluded that people with a high trans-fatty acid level had a three times higher risk of sudden cardiac death than people with lower levels.

Found in over 42,000 food products, trans fat is hard to avoid. While the average American consumes close to 5 grams of the substance a day, researchers say even one gram – which can drive up LDL cholesterol levels – is too much in a healthy diet. According to Alice Lichtenstein, a nutritional biochemist at Tufts University, if you double the amount of trans fat you eat, you nearly double your LDL cholesterol.

The major sources of trans fatty acids come from partially hydrogenated vegetable fat, which is used for commercial frying,

---

HEART SMART TIP
Just Say No To Trans Fats

While trans fat is used to make cookies, crackers and chips, much of this phony fat in our diet comes from margarine. Does that mean you should buy one of the new "trans fat free" spreads? Absolutely not! These margarines are still manmade plastics that the body was never designed to handle.

Butter, in small amounts, is a better option. Although high in saturated fat, butter is a rich source of vitamins A and D, as well as trace minerals like selenium. For cooking, choose either ghee (clarified butter available in health food stores) or extra-virgin olive oil. A recent study found that ghee actually helps the body digest dietary fat, especially if you are also taking a fish oil supplement. Other research has found that olive oil decreases oxidative stress. But remember, these are still fats, so use them sparingly.

says Lichtenstein. Trans fat can also be found in commercial baked goods, frozen foods, candy, crackers and even ready-to-eat breakfast cereal.

The problem is, there's no way to know for sure if the food you're buying contains trans fats. Even food labeled "low in cholesterol" or "low in saturated fats" may contain large amounts of trans fats. Beginning in 2006, all ingredient labels will be required to list the amount of trans fat in foods. But in the meantime, if you see the word 'hydrogenated' on a food label, you can assume it contains trans fatty acids.

Eat Like A Greek – Or Maybe An Asian

Maybe you've heard that the rate of heart disease is uncommonly low among people living in the Mediterranean. The reason is simple. Unlike those of us in U.S., these folks eat lots of vegetables, fruits, grains and olive oil. And, while most Americans have come to embrace the benefits of olive oil, it's not the only thing that makes the Mediterranean diet heart healthy.

In the largest study ever done on the Mediterranean diet, and one of the few to test it in adults of all ages, researchers recently found that the real bang of this way of eating is the combination of all the foods in the diet. Not surprisingly, the researchers found that Greeks who follow the Mediterranean diet more closely have significantly lower death and disease rates than those who don't. But they also reported in *The New England Journal of Medicine* that olive oil itself produced no significant reduction in overall death rates. In fact, when the researchers looked at the individual components of the Mediterranean diet, they found no significant decrease in death with any one type of food.

The researchers studied some 22,000 adults, aged 20 to 86, from all regions of Greece. The participants answered detailed questionnaires about their eating habits throughout the four-year study. Then they were rated on how closely they followed the key principles of the Mediterranean diet. Sticking to the Mediterranean diet cut the risk of death from both heart disease and cancer. Those subjects who most closely followed the traditional diet saw their death rate drop by 25 percent.

Asians also enjoy unprecedented heart health. Like the Mediterranean diet, they eat high amounts of grains and vegetables. But the real secret to their cardiovascular health is fish. Most recent studies have shown that people who eat fish at least once a week have a 60 percent lower risk of heart disease than those who rarely eat fish. Case in point: In Lisbon, Portugal, scientists compared the differences in heart disease between a fishing village and an inland rural village on the island of Madeira. The results were startling. Death rates from heart disease in the fishing village were a mere 310 in 100,000 men compared to more than 1,200 in 100,000 in the rural village.

Closer to home, researchers at the University of Oregon found that volunteers who ate salmon every day for four weeks experienced a 17 percent drop in their cholesterol and a 40 percent reduction in triglycerides. The Oregon team also found that high fish consumption lowered the risk of atherosclerosis by preventing platelets from sticking together. These findings were confirmed by a double-blind, placebo-controlled trial at Massachusetts General Hospital in Boston, which found that small amounts of fish oil – the kind found in salmon and tuna – inhibit platelet aggregation and lower triglycerides. Even more interesting, the fish oil appeared to significantly reduce systolic blood pressure by as much as 8 mmHg.

There is also some evidence that the omega-3 fatty acids in fish can tame C-reactive protein. *The American Journal of Cardiology* reports that, among 269 cardiac patients, those who had the highest serum concentration of DHA (short for docosahexaenoic acid, an important omega-3 fatty acid) as a result of eating fish on a regular basis also had less risk for coronary stenosis (the narrowing of the blood vessels).

I strongly recommend eating fatty fish at least three times a week. The best sources of omega-3 fatty acids are salmon, tuna, mackerel, herring, sardines, anchovies and trout. But be aware that tuna can harbor unacceptable levels of mercury and shouldn't be eaten more than once a week. This toxic heavy metal accumulates in the flesh of fish and can build up in people who eat more than two servings of fish a week. Mercury has been linked to neurological disorders, kidney damage and atherosclerosis. I think all patients with heart disease should be screened for mercury. Common methods include blood tests,

HEART SMART TIP
Feast On Fish

Need to lower CRP? While aspirin can lower this marker of inflammation, it can also cause bleeding, ulcers and low prostaglandins. And, while statin drugs may have a mild effect on CRP, they destroy Co-Q10.

What to do? Include fatty fish in your diet at least three times a week – or take supplemental fish oil. Best choices: Salmon, tuna or trout.

SAFETY ALERT!

While salmon is relatively low in mercury, if you buy farm-raised salmon, you might be getting more than you paid for. According to a new scientific report, salmon from fish farms has significantly higher levels of polychlorinated biphenyl (PCBs) than wild Pacific salmon. PCBs, which lodge in fatty tissue, were banned in the U.S. in the late-1970s because they can cause cancer and birth defects.

To reduce your exposure to PCBs, choose wild or canned Alaskan salmon instead of farmed whenever possible. If farm-raised salmon is unavoidable, limit your consumption to once a month. Trim the fat and skin from the fish before cooking and avoid frying. Broiling, baking or grilling allows the PCB-laden fat to cook off the fish.

measuring urinary excretion or hair analysis and I strongly advise asking your doctor to schedule you for these simple tests.

Up Your Antioxidants

Other villains in the development of heart disease are free radicals. Free radicals are molecules that are missing one electron (normal molecules have two electrons). To complete themselves, these unbalanced molecules steal a replacement electron from another nearby molecule – which creates another free radical, which steals an electron from one of its neighbors and so on and so on. The result is a chain reaction that can ultimately damage DNA, proteins and other cellular building blocks.

Free radicals play a big role in the development of atherosclerosis. The process of plaque build-up begins when free radicals damage the wall of the artery, causing a lesion. In an attempt to repair the damage, white blood cells called monocytes come to the rescue. Once they enter the artery walls, these monocytes are converted into macrophages that gobble up fat and cholesterol, especially LDL cholesterol. Think of it as a biological Pac Man game.

The problem is that, once these macrophages are loaded up with LDL, they get stuck in the cell walls. Worse yet, macrophages can also generate free radicals. The result is a build-up of atherosclerotic plaque. The good news is that we can counteract much of this damage – as well as our risk of premature aging and disease – with antioxidants.

For years, scientists have known that antioxidants can neutralize these unruly molecules and prevent oxidative damage. And for years, they've been studying them – one at a time. But by studying each individual antioxidant in the hope of finding a magic bullet, they've missed the bigger picture – that antioxidants never occur by themselves in nature. A strawberry, for instance, doesn't contain just one antioxidant. It's packed full of vitamin C, carotenoids and flavonoids.

A growing number of important studies have concluded that antioxidants work in synergy. In other words, consuming a combination of many different antioxidants is far more potent than taking just one or two. Here's a good example: as vitamin E is used up fighting free radicals, vitamin C helps restore it back to its full strength.

One study, recently published in the journal *Atherosclerosis*, found that a combination of vitamin E and C significantly reduce the formation of plaque after an angioplasty. In another clinical trial of 23 patients with coronary artery disease, Chilean researchers found that taking supplemental beta-carotene and vitamins E and C can reduce serum homocystine levels and LDL (bad) cholesterol oxidation.

Antioxidants also play a role after a heart attack. A double-blind, placebo controlled study of 125 patients tested the therapeutic value of antioxidants in reducing complications after a heart attack. At the end of the study, the scientists concluded that combined treatment with vitamins A, C, E and beta-carotene helped protect heart attack victims against angina and oxidative stress as they recovered. Better yet, the antioxidants seemed to lower the risk of another cardiac event.

Nature's antioxidants can never be replaced by simply popping a few pills, so you should always strive to include a wide variety of fruits and vegetables every day. These foods contain a more diverse selection of antioxidants than you'll find in any supplement. And that's one reason why a diet rich in these foods lowers your risk of just about every degenerative disease.

Fuel Up On Fiber

Fiber may just be the unsung hero of heart health. According to a joint study by Brigham and Women's Hospital and Harvard

Medical School, boosting your fiber intake can significantly reduce the risk of cardiovascular disease and heart attack. Dietary fiber lowers LDL and homocystine levels, as well as blood pressure. Fiber also decreases the incidence of blood clots that may cause heart attacks and strokes.

Unfortunately, the average American diet contains only half of the recommended 25 to 35 grams of fiber you should be consuming daily to promote health. But before you stock up on fiber-rich foods, there are a couple of things you need to know.

Fiber is the portion of plant food that human digestive enzymes can't break down and there are two major types – insoluble and soluble. Insoluble fiber is a "non-carbohydrate" carbohydrate that passes through the gastrointestinal tract undigested. Unlike soluble fiber, insoluble fibers aren't metabolized by intestinal bacteria. Good sources of insoluble fiber are: corn, popcorn, the skins of many fruits and vegetables, seeds, nuts and whole grains.

Soluble fiber is that part of the plant that can be absorbed into the body. About one-quarter of the total fiber in food is the soluble type. Oats, beans and other legumes, and some fruits and vegetables are all good sources of soluble fiber. Flaxseeds, which are high in heart-healthy omega-3 fatty acids, are another source of soluble fiber.

Both types of fiber can help you achieve and maintain your ideal weight and provide benefits to the

Sources of Soluble Fiber

Barley	Parsnips
Flaxseeds	Sweet Potatoes
Oatmeal	Turnips
Oat Bran	Apples
Dried Beans	Figs
Lentils	Kiwi Fruit
Lima Beans	Mangos
Chickpeas	Oranges
Brussels Sprouts	Plums
Artichokes	Prunes

digestive system by helping to maintain regularity. But soluble fiber has some additional benefits to heart health. Soluble fiber reduces cholesterol by binding to bile acids and whisking them out of the body. This type of fiber also slows down the production of cholesterol in the liver – much like bile-sequestering agents. Adding just 5 to 10 grams of soluble fiber to your diet every day can reduce cholesterol levels by five points – which translates to a 10 percent drop in the risk of heart disease.

Here's a good illustration of just how effective soluble fiber is: According to researchers at Tulane University, adding legumes (beans and peas) to your diet on a regular basis can significantly lower the risk of heart disease. After analyzing the data from their 19-year study of more than 9,600 volunteers, the researchers found that those who ate beans four times a week or more had a 22 percent lower risk of heart disease than the volunteers who only ate legumes once a week.

HEART SMART TIP
Say Nuts to Heart Disease!

Nuts are a great source of vitamin E and healthy fats that help lower cholesterol levels. And they are full of soluble fiber. According to the Physician's Health Study, nuts also contain compounds with anti-arrhythmic properties which may reduce sudden cardiac death. So add at least two handfuls of nuts per week to your diet, especially walnuts or almonds. But eat them raw since roasting destroys their delicate polyunsaturated fats.

If you're not getting enough fiber through your diet, you can take a psyllium supplement, available in powder, capsule or tablet form. Mixed with at least eight ounces of water, psyllium expands tenfold in your digestive tract to thwart cholesterol. The secret to making fiber supplements work, however, is water – lots of it. If you use a fiber supplement, make sure to drink at least 10 glasses of water a day.

The Joy of Soy

Over the last decade, soy has become a kitchen staple for many health-conscious Americans. No wonder – soy is high in protein, low in fat and excellent source of fiber, calcium, the B vitamins and omega-3 fatty acids.

If that isn't enough to send you straight to the soy aisle of your supermarket, the American Heart Association credits soy protein with lowering both total and LDL cholesterol. The AHA bases its endorsement on more than 40 studies which show that either adding soy protein to your diet or replacing animal protein with soy can:

√ Decrease serum LDL levels by 12.9 percent

√ Lower serum triglyceride levels by 10.5 percent

√ Increase HDL levels slightly

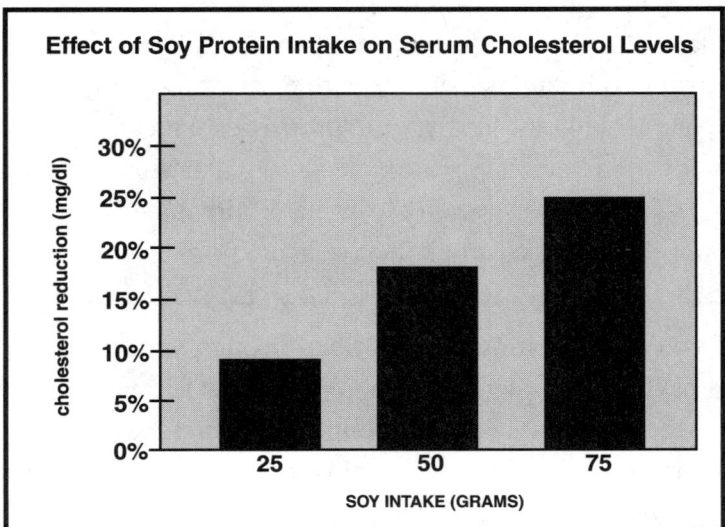

But to accomplish this, you need to consume at least 25 grams of soy protein a day, which is equivalent to two glasses of soy milk or a half a pound of tofu. As the chart on the previous page illustrates, adding just 25 grams of soy protein to your diet every day can reduce cholesterol by nearly 10 percent. But, as you can see, when it comes to soy, more is definitely better.

Soy contains several compounds that boost heart health – specifically isoflavones, saponins and phytosterols. Here's what makes each of them such stellar protectors of your heart:

- *Isoflavones* are potent antioxidants that can help neutralize free radicals. One particularly effective isoflavone is genistein, which discourages the formation of potentially dangerous blood clots.

- *Saponins* bind to cholesterol in the gastrointestinal tract so that it isn't absorbed by the intestines. The cholesterol then passes directly to the colon where it is excreted from the body.

- *Phytosterols* lower cholesterol levels by inhibiting absorption. Studies have found that plant sterol and stanol esters can lower cholesterol by 10 to 14 percent.

Soyfood	Grams of protein
Soybeans, 1/2 cup cooked	14
Soymilk, 1 cup	7
Roasted soy nuts, 1/2 cup	34
Soy flour, 1/4 cup	8
Tempeh, 1/2 cup	16
TVP, 1/2 cup prepared	11
Tofu, 1/2 cup	10

Including soy in your diet is easy. In addition to traditional tofu, grocery stores now offer an incredibly wide variety of soy foods.

Look for soy burgers, soy milk, soy yogurt, soy cheese and soy nuts. As soy becomes a staple in your diet, try some tempeh or TVP. Tempeh is a fermented soy product with a nutty mushroom flavor and a great addition to soups, spreads, salads and sandwiches. TVP, which stands for textured vegetable protein, is a dried soy-based meat substitute that can be used in place of ground meat in chili, spaghetti sauce, tacos or casseroles.

Glorious Garlic

Garlic is another great food for your heart. Recent studies suggest that this tasty herb can reduce the build-up of plaque in the arteries. There is also evidence that garlic lowers blood pressure and protects against free radical damage. Even more important, garlic helps to improve the ratio of LDL and HDL. I'll tell you more about garlic's medicinal properties in Chapter 9. Meanwhile, make a conscious effort to include more garlic in the dishes you create.

The Coffee Question

If you're like most people, your day probably starts sometime after your first cup of coffee. Yet studies show that the caffeine in coffee activates the sympathetic nervous system, which increases your heart rate and blood pressure. Concerns have also been raised that high caffeine intake may boost homocystine levels. In fact, a recent study by Dutch researchers found that brewed coffee increased homocystine levels by 11 percent within hours of consumption, and seemed to have a particularly strong effect when taken after meals.

Instead of coffee, try switching to tea. According to new research from the U.S. Department of Agriculture, regularly drinking black tea may lower cholesterol levels. In the six-week trial that included 15 participants, nearly half drank five cups of black tea daily for three weeks. The investigators gave the other subjects colored water that was flavored like tea. The two groups were then switched, and the subjects received either the placebo drink or black tea for another three weeks. By the end of the study, the researchers discovered that LDL cholesterol dropped an average of 7.5 percent during the three weeks the participants consumed black tea compared with the placebo drink.

Earlier research also found that people who drank 12 ounces or more of black tea a day had more than 50 percent fewer heart attacks. In one study, researchers at Tufts University examined 1,900 heart-attack victims. They found that those who drank the most tea before their first heart attack were 44 percent less likely to die during the following three to four years.

Green tea may be even better. This Japanese staple is extremely high in antioxidants, which fights free radical damage and may reduce the stickiness of platelets. Recent research has also found that green tea may help the body regulate LDL cholesterol. But to get the benefits, you need to drink at least three cups of green tea a day.

Go Easy on Alcohol

Occasional drinkers may have fewer heart attacks and strokes than abstainers and those who drink more heavily. That's because a little alcohol can raise levels of good HDL cholesterol and can reduce the risk of heart attack and stroke by helping prevent blood clots in the arteries.

But if you're looking to lower cholesterol, opt for red wine. Cabernet Sauvignon, Merlot, red Zinfandel and other red wines contain two compounds that can reign in cholesterol levels. The first is one you may have heard of: Resveratrol. Several studies have found that resveratrol blocks cholesterol oxidation. The second is a class of compounds known as saponins. Researchers at the University of California-Davis recently found these compounds bind to and prevent the absorption of cholesterol.

The watchword in all of this, of course, is moderation. For men, that means fewer than two drinks a day. Women should limit themselves to no more than one drink a day. People who drink alcohol in amounts that exceed the limits of moderation have higher death rates than do moderate drinkers, primarily from liver disease, high blood pressure, alcohol-related heart diseases and some types of cancer.

Now that you know what foods to eat, make sure you aren't undermining your efforts – buy only the freshest, most unadulterated foods available. Much of what is on grocery store shelves harbors pesticide residue and chemical additives. And a growing number of foods have been genetically modified. Dubbed "frankenfoods" by critics, the long-term safety of consuming these foods has not been established.

Protect yourself from harmful chemicals and dubious science by eating organic foods as often as possible. Organic foods offer a safe and sustainable food supply. Better yet, researchers are finding evidence that organically-grown produce contains more nutrients than conventionally grown plants.

Diet Do's and Don'ts

Admittedly, switching to a heart-healthy diet requires some adjustment. Here are a few tips to help you make the transition:

- Eat a variety of fruits and vegetables – at least three servings of each a day.

- Pass up refined breads and pastas in favor of whole grains.

- Avoid convenience foods and commercially-baked goods.

- Switch to low-fat or fat-free dairy products.

- Choose and prepare foods with less salt. For additional flavor, add herbs, spices or lemon juice.

- Substitute Bragg Liquid Aminos for tamari or soy sauce.

- Steer clear of fried foods. Roasting, steaming, poaching and broiling are much healthier alternatives.

- Instead of using oil, try sautéing in a bit of water, stock or wine.

- If you must use oil, opt for extra virgin olive oil or organic canola oil and use as little as possible.

- Instead of fat-filled commercial salad dressings, make your own using olive or flaxseed oil, flavored vinegars and herbs.

- Substitute mustard or fat-free salad dressing for mayonnaise on sandwiches.

- Eat more fish and lean poultry. Just remember to remove the skin and all visible fat from chicken before cooking.

- Replace the milk called for in recipes with plain soymilk.

- If you're suffering from a snack attack, try frozen fruit or fiber-rich popcorn. But instead of salt, try adding chili powder or cumin. And forget the butter.

- Eat more nuts – but opt for raw nuts instead of the roasted, salted varieties.

Heart Healthy Recipes

Adopting a heart-smart diet can be fun and delicious. Think of it as cardiovascular creativity. If you need some help putting your new diet together, there are a number of cookbooks on the market that offer recipes, menus and cooking tips specifically created to promote heart health. In fact, gourmet guru Graham Kerr has even written one!

To get you started on a heart-healthy eating plan, here are 25 of my favorite recipes. All are low in sodium, saturated fat and cholesterol. But more importantly, these recipes contain high levels of fiber, antioxidants and beneficial fats. Unless otherwise noted, these easy-to-prepare recipes contain ingredients available at your local grocery store. And feel free to substitute canned for dried beans.

However, since processing can destroy some of the nutrients found in beans, it's best to soak and cook them yourself if you have time. Another bonus – dried beans are less expensive than their canned counterparts!

Breakfast

♥

Garden Omelet

Serves 2

Try this sumptuous omelet for a leisurely Sunday brunch.

1/2 cup mushrooms, sliced
1/2 cup onions, chopped
1/4 cup red bell pepper, chopped
1 cup fresh spinach, chopped
1-1/2 teaspoon olive oil, divided
4 egg whites
2 whole eggs
4 teaspoons water
1/4 teaspoon salt
Dash pepper
1/2 cup Monterey jack-style soy cheese, shredded

Heat one teaspoon of olive oil in a skillet. Add the vegetables and sauté until just tender. Remove from pan and keep warm. In a medium bowl, whisk together the eggs, water, salt and pepper. Heat the remaining oil in the skillet. Pour half of the egg mixture into the pan, tilting to coat the bottom. Gently lift the edges to allow the uncooked egg to slide underneath the omelet. When all of the egg has cooked, slide onto a plate. Add half of the vegetables and 1/4 cup of the cheese to one half of the omelet. Carefully fold over. Repeat with the remaining eggs, vegetables and cheese.

Tofu Scramble

Serves 6

Who says you have to give up scrambled eggs? By substituting tofu, you can enjoy this breakfast standby – minus the cholesterol!

1 small onion, chopped
1/2 cup green pepper, chopped
1/2 cup mushrooms, sliced
1 teaspoon olive oil
2 cups firm tofu, drained and crumbled
1 tablespoon Bragg Liquid Aminos
1 teaspoon parsley flakes
1/2 teaspoon turmeric
Dash pepper

Using a large skillet, sauté the vegetables in the olive oil. Add the remaining ingredients and stir to mix well. Cook for five minutes, stirring frequently to prevent sticking.

Very Berry Smoothie

Serves 2

Packed with antioxidants, this delicious "breakfast-in-a-glass" is perfect on a busy morning. Using fresh organic fruit is best, but you can substitute frozen fruit if desired.

1 cup vanilla-flavored soy yogurt
1/2 cup strawberries
1/2 cup raspberries
1/2 cup blackberries
1/2 cup blueberries
1/4 cup maple syrup

Place all of the ingredients in a blender and blend until thick and creamy. If the smoothie becomes too thick to blend, add a bit of vanilla soy milk.

Soups & Salads
♥

Mellow Miso Soup

Serves 6

This traditional Japanese soup is as nutritious as it is delicious.
Look for the seaweed and dashi powder in Asian markets.

1/2 teaspoon dried kombu seaweed
4 dried shiitake mushrooms
8 cups water
1 envelope dashi powder
1/3 cup red miso, or to taste
2 green onions, sliced

Over high heat, bring the water to a rolling boil. Reduce heat and add the kombu and mushrooms. Cover and simmer for about 45 minutes. Remove the kombu and mushrooms and set aside to cool. Add half of the dashi powder to the pot and stir. Simmer for 10-15 minutes. Meanwhile, slice the kombu and mushrooms. Add the miso, kombu and mushrooms to the broth and remove from heat. Garnish with sliced green onions.

Lemony Lentil Soup

Serves 6

This hearty soup offers up a hefty serving of protein, fiber,
vitamin A, folate, calcium and potassium. Its earthy flavor is
brightened with a twist of sprightly lemon.

1 cup brown lentils
6 cups fat-free, low-sodium chicken broth
2-1/2 cups water
1 large onion, chopped
Pinch crushed red pepper
4 cloves garlic, minced

1 bunch Swiss chard, ribs removed and leaves chopped
1/2 cup cilantro, chopped
1/3 cup fresh lemon juice

In a medium saucepan, combine the lentils with the stock and two cups of the water. Bring to a boil. Reduce the heat, cover and simmer until the lentils are barely tender, about 30 minutes.

Meanwhile, heat the remaining half-cup of water in a large skillet over medium heat. Add the onions, crushed pepper and garlic, stirring to prevent sticking, until the onion is lightly browned. Gradually add the chard and additional water, if needed, stirring occasionally until wilted.

Add the chard mixture to the lentils. Cover and simmer for 15 minutes. Just before serving, add the cilantro and lemon juice. Stir well and serve.

"Heart-y" Minestrone Soup

Serves 6

Don't let the long list of ingredients fool you. This quick main-dish soup couldn't be easier – or healthier!

1 15-ounce can kidney beans
1 15-ounce can garbanzo beans
1 onion, chopped
3 cloves garlic, minced
8 cups water
1/2 cup celery, thinly sliced
1 carrot, peeled and sliced
1 cup green beans, cut into 1-inch pieces
1 8-ounce can low-sodium tomato sauce
1 15-ounce can crushed tomatoes
1/4 cup parsley, chopped
2 teaspoons dried basil
1-1/2 teaspoons dried oregano

1/4 teaspoon pepper
1 zucchini, chopped
1 cup cabbage, shredded
1 10-ounce package frozen chopped spinach
1/2 cup whole-wheat elbow macaroni

Drain and rinse the beans. Place the beans, onions, garlic and water in a Dutch oven. Heat to boiling, reduce heat and simmer for 20 minutes. Add the celery, carrot, green beans, tomato sauce, crushed tomatoes, parsley, basil, oregano and pepper. Continue to simmer for an additional 30 minutes. Add the zucchini, cabbage, spinach and macaroni. Cook until tender, approximately 20 minutes.

Asian Kale Salad

Serves 4

This unusual salad is a terrific source of both vitamins A and C, as well as calcium.

1 bunch kale, roughly chopped
1 bunch romaine hearts, roughly chopped
1/2 red onion, thinly sliced
1/4 cup seasoned rice wine vinegar
1 teaspoon pureed ginger
1/2 teaspoon light sesame oil
5 drops dark sesame oil
1 teaspoon honey
1 teaspoon Bragg Liquid Aminos

Combine the kale, romaine and onions in a salad bowl. Using a blender, blend the remaining ingredients until thoroughly mixed. Pour over salad and toss well. (Note: You can substitute bottled dressing, such as Annie's Natural's Shiitake & Sesame Vinaigrette, if desired.)

Tex-Mex Black Bean Salad

Serves 6

An excellent source of protein and vitamins A, C and the B vitamins. This salad is a wonderful dish to bring to potlucks. Everyone loves it!

2 cans black beans, drained and rinsed
1 cup frozen corn kernels, defrosted
1/2 red onion, chopped
1/4 cup olive oil
1/4 cup flaxseed oil
1/4 cup balsamic vinegar
1/2 teaspoon dried basil
2 cloves garlic, minced
1/8 teaspoon pepper

   In a large bowl, mix all ingredients except lettuce leaves. Refrigerate for at least 30 minutes. Line a platter or bowl with lettuce leaves and spoon the bean salad into the serving dish.

Tabouli

Serves 4

Light and tangy, this refreshing salad is perfect for a summer lunch. As a bonus, this dish is high in fiber and vitamin A, with respectable quantities of folate, calcium and magnesium.

1 cup bulgur
2 cups boiling water
2 tomatoes, diced
1 bunch green onions, sliced
3 tablespoons fresh mint, chopped
2 cups parsley, chopped
1/2 cup fresh lemon juice
1/4 cup olive oil
Pepper to taste

Place uncooked bulgur in a bowl; pour water over it and let it soak one hour, stirring occasionally. Drain well in a fine strainer. Return the bulgur to the bowl and add all other ingredients; mix well. Chill least 2 hours before serving.

A Better Waldorf Salad

Serves 6

Forget the heavy, mayonnaise-laden salad of yesteryear. This low-fat version combines plenty of fiber with heart-healthy fats.

5 cups unpeeled apples, cored and chopped
1 cup celery, diced
1/2 cup walnuts, chopped
1/2 cup raisins
1/2 teaspoon lemon juice
1/2 cup plain yogurt
2 tablespoons honey
1 tablespoon pineapple juice

Mix the first 5 ingredients in a large bowl. In another bowl, whisk together remaining ingredients. Pour the dressing over fruit mixture and stir until evenly coated. Cover and chill 30 minutes before serving to give the flavors a chance to mingle. Toss again before serving.

Sandwiches & Spreads

♥

Harvest Sandwich

Serves 1

This fiber-rich sandwich is wonderful when gardens and farmer's markets are overflowing with fresh produce. It's also a tasty way to include raw veggies in your diet.

2 slices whole wheat bread
2 tablespoons fat-free Italian salad dressing
Any combination of the following:
Sliced red onions
Sliced tomatoes
Sliced cucumbers
Sliced radishes
Sliced green pepper
Shredded carrot
Spinach leaves
Lettuce leaves
Alfalfa sprouts

Spread each slice of bread with the dressing. Layer the vegetables on one slice and top with the remaining slice.

Herbed Bean & Cucumber Sandwich

Serves 4

Keep this creamy, fiber-filled spread in your refrigerator for a quick and tasty lunch.

1 cup canned white beans
2 tablespoons parsley, chopped
1 tablespoon green onion, sliced
1 teaspoon dill weed
1/4 teaspoon salt

Pepper, to taste
2 ounces light cream cheese
1 tablespoon lemon juice
8 slices whole grain bread
1 cucumber, peeled and thinly sliced
Lettuce leaves
Broccoli or alfalfa sprouts

Combine beans, herbs, salt, pepper, cheese and lemon juice in a food processor and process until smooth. Spread the mixture on four slices of bread. Top with the remaining ingredients and close the sandwiches.

Lentil Burgers

Serves 12

This low-fat recipe makes 12 patties, so freeze the leftovers for the next time you're in the mood for burgers.

1 cup lentils
3 cups water, divided
1 bay leaf
1/2 cup onion, diced
1 tablespoons fresh tarragon, chopped
2 teaspoons fresh marjoram, chopped
1 teaspoon ground cumin
1/2 teaspoon dark sesame oil
1/2 teaspoon lemon juice
1/2 teaspoon salt
1/4 teaspoon pepper
3/4 cup rolled oats
3/4 cup whole-grain bread crumbs

In a medium saucepan, combine the lentils with 2-1/2 cups of water and simmer for about 45 minutes, or until the lentils are tender. Drain well and return to pan.

Meanwhile, sauté the onion in the remaining water until lightly browned. Remove from heat and stir in the herbs and spices. Add the onion mixture to the lentils and stir until thoroughly combined.

Process the oats in a blender or food processor until finely ground. Add the oats and bread crumbs to the lentils, mixing well. Shape the mixture into 12 patties.

Preheat the oven to 400°F. Bake the patties on a non-stick baking sheet until the patties are lightly browned, about 15 minutes. Serve on whole-grain buns.

Hummus

Serves 4

This middle-eastern spread is great to have on hand for snacks, sandwiches or dips.

2-1/2 cups canned garbanzo beans, drained and rinsed
1/4 cup lemon juice
Vegetable broth
6 cloves garlic, roasted
1 clove garlic, minced
Zest of one lemon
1/2 teaspoon cumin
1/2 teaspoon coriander
1/8 teaspoon cayenne pepper
Salt to taste

Place the beans and lemon juice in a food processor and puree. While the machine is running, add enough vegetable broth to form a creamy texture. Continue to puree as you add the remaining ingredients. Scoop into an airtight container and chill for at least one hour. Serve with whole wheat pita triangles or raw vegetables. (Note: for variation, add 1/4 cup of roasted red pepper to the mixture while processing.)

Entrees
♥

Honey-Citrus Glazed Salmon

Serves 4

This savory dish is an excellent source of omega-3 fatty acids.

Cooking spray
4 salmon filets
1/4 cup orange juice
1 teaspoon orange zest, grated
1 tablespoon honey
1/2 teaspoon cumin
1 green onion, sliced

Preheat oven to 400°F. Lightly coat a baking sheet with cooking spray.

In a shallow dish, whisk together orange juice, zest, honey and cumin. Add salmon and turn to coat. Allow the fish to marinate for 10 to 15 minutes.

Transfer the salmon to the prepared baking sheet and brush with marinade. Bake for 10 minutes or until the fish flakes easily with a fork. Garnish with green onions and serve.

Asian Grilled Ahi

Serves 4

This mouth-watering dish is a great source of omega-3 fatty acids and selenium. But don't indulge too often. Tuna is high in mercury, so limit your intake.

4 1-inch thick ahi tuna steaks
2 teaspoons olive oil
Lots of freshly ground pepper
1 teaspoon canola oil
2 tablespoons fresh ginger, peeled and minced

2 tablespoons Bragg Liquid Aminos

1 tablespoon brown sugar

1/4 cup water

1/2 teaspoon dark sesame oil

Rub each tuna steak with a small amount of olive oil and season generously with pepper. Preheat the grill. Meanwhile, prepare the sauce: Sauté the ginger in the canola oil for a minute or two. Add the remaining ingredients and simmer for 5 minutes. Remove from heat.

Grill the tuna for 2-3 minutes on each side. Serve with the sauce on the side.

Chicken Corazón

Serves 4

A good source of low-fat protein, this main dish is low in cholesterol and high in flavor.

1/3 cup lime juice

1/4 cup Bragg Liquid Aminos

1 teaspoon olive oil

1-1/2 teaspoons chili powder

1-1/2 teaspoons cumin

1-1/2 teaspoons coriander

1/4 teaspoon turmeric

6 cloves garlic, minced

1-1/2 teaspoons honey

1/4 cup white wine

1/4 cup cilantro, chopped

4 skinless, boneless chicken breasts, trimmed of all fat

Mix together the first 11 ingredients in a large baking pan. Add the chicken and turn to coat. Cover and refrigerate for at least two hours.

Preheat the broiler. Broil the chicken for 8 to 10 minutes,

basting with the marinade every few minutes. Garnish with cilantro sprigs and serve with salsa.

Penne Pomodoro

Serves 4

Brimming with fresh tomatoes and basil, this pasta is packed with lycopene and reservatrol.

6 cloves garlic, minced
1/2 cup red onion, chopped
1/2 cup water
6 roma tomatoes, chopped
1 cup red wine
1 bunch fresh basil, chopped
12 ounces penne pasta
Freshly grated parmesan cheese

Sauté garlic and onions in the water until the onions are well browned. Add the tomatoes and sauté until they begin to break down. Stir in the red wine and bring to a boil. Reduce heat and simmer for 15 minutes. Add the basil and simmer for an additional 5 minutes. Meanwhile, boil the pasta. When the pasta is al dente, drain and return to pot. Mix the sauce with the pasta, tossing well to coat. Serve with a sprinkling of parmesan cheese.

Whole Bean Chili

Serves 4

This meatless chili is high in folate and lycopene.
Feel free to adjust the spices to suit your taste.

2 cups dried kidney beans
5 cups water
2 onions, chopped
1 green pepper, chopped

3 cloves garlic, minced

1 cup low-sodium tomato sauce

1 15-ounce can low-sodium stewed tomatoes

4 tablespoons chili powder

2 teaspoons cumin

1/4 teaspoon crushed red pepper

1/4 teaspoon turmeric

Soak the beans overnight. Place the beans and water in a Dutch oven. Bring to a boil, then reduce the heat to low. Cover and simmer for 1 hour. Add the remaining ingredients and stir to mix well. Cover and simmer for an additional 2 hours, stirring occasionally. Ladle into bowls and garnish with my antioxidant-rich onion blend. (Note: For an extra dose of fiber, serve over brown rice.)

To make the onion blend: Sauté 2 cloves of freshly minced garlic, one-quarter sliced Vidalia onion and one sliced shiitake mushroom in one teaspoon of olive oil. Season to taste with pepper and/or turmeric. (Note: this mixture is also wonderful on steamed or sautéed vegetables.)

Warming Winter Stew

Serves 6

Hearty and healthy, this vegetarian stew is packed with heart-healthy fiber, vitamins A and C, folate, iron, and B vitamins. This versatile stew is open to interpretation, so feel free to add or substitute different vegetables for the ones listed below. Tasty options include zucchini, parsnips or Swiss chard.

1 cup lentils, rinsed
4 cups vegetable broth
1 cup water
2 cups sweet potato, peeled and cubed
1/2 cup onion, chopped
1/2 cup celery, sliced
2 cloves garlic, minced
2 teaspoons Bragg Liquid Aminos
2 teaspoons cumin
1 teaspoon coriander
1/2 teaspoon turmeric
1 15-ounce can garbanzo beans
1 1/2 cups green beans
1 1/2 cups broccoli florets
2 green onions, sliced (optional)

In a large pot or Dutch oven, combine lentils with broth and bring to a boil. Reduce the heat and simmer until lentils are barely tender, 20 to 30 minutes. Add the water, sweet potato, onion, celery, garlic, Bragg Liquid Aminos and spices, and cook partially covered for about 40 minutes on medium heat. Add more broth or water if soup seems too thick. Add the garbanzo beans, green beans and broccoli. Simmer for 15 minutes. Garnish with green onions, if desired.

Grilled Summer Vegetables

Serves 2

Satisfying and full of antioxidants. Serve with a whole-grain pilaf for a complete meal.

2 portobello mushrooms

2 zucchini

2 yellow squash

2 red peppers

10 asparagus spears

1/4 cup olive oil

1/4 cup flaxseed oil

1/4 cup balsamic vinegar

1/2 tsp. dried basil

2 cloves garlic, minced

1/8 tsp. pepper

Remove stem and lightly wash mushrooms. Wash and cut the zucchini and yellow squash lengthwise into 1/4-inch slices. Cut the red peppers in half and remove seeds and stem. Rinse the asparagus. Set all vegetables aside.

To make the marinade: Combine the remaining ingredients in a blender and blend to mix. Place the vegetables in a large Ziploc bag and add the marinade. Marinate for 30 minutes.

Meanwhile, preheat the grill. Drain the vegetables, reserving marinade, and grill over medium heat for 4-5 minutes, keeping a constant watch to prevent burning. Turn and grill for an additional 2-3 minutes. Arrange on a large platter and garnish with fresh parsley or green onions. Serve reserved marinade in a separate bowl for dipping.

HEART SMART TIP
Get Sweet Without The Sugar

Several years ago, doctors at Chicago's Rush Medical College recommended that patients with high triglycerides avoid refined sugar. It's not the first time researchers have linked sugar to heart disease. What's the alternative? Use honey or stevia (an herb that's 300 times sweeter than sugar and calorie free!)

As a general rule, use half to 2/3 as much honey as sugar and reduce the liquid in the recipe by 1/4 cup for each cup of honey used. If you are using stevia, substitute 1 teaspoon of liquid or powdered stevia for each cup of sugar.

Desserts

❤

Sparkling Berries

Serves 4

This light, refreshing dessert packs a potent nutritional punch. High in vitamins A and C, folate, calcium and potassium, it's the perfect way to celebrate summer's berry season.

1/2 cup fresh strawberries, sliced
1/2 cup fresh blueberries
1/2 cup fresh raspberries
1/2 cup fresh blackberries
Sparkling water

Gently combine the berries in a bowl until well mixed. Spoon into tall goblets or champagne flutes. Just before serving, pour sparkling water over the berries to fill each goblet.

Blueberry Cinnamon Compote

Serves 4

*This is delicious on its own or spooned over
soy-based vanilla ice cream.*

3 cups blueberries
1 tablespoon lemon juice
1 teaspoon lemon peel, grated
1/2 teaspoon cinnamon
3/4 cup sugar

Combine all the ingredients in a medium saucepan and
simmer over medium heat for 5 minutes, stirring to dissolve sugar.
Serve warm or allow to cool to room temperature.

Honey Baked Apples

Serves 4

*Apples are one of Mother Nature's original health foods. This
fiber-rich dessert is a smart way to satisfy your sweet-tooth.*

1-1/2 cups apple juice
1/4 cup lemon juice
4 tablespoons honey
1/2 teaspoon cinnamon
2 tablespoons raisins
4 baking apples

Preheat the oven to 400°F. In a small saucepan, combine all of
the ingredients except the raisins and apples. Bring to a boil,
stirring constantly, until the mixture has thickened. Remove from
heat and stir in the raisins.

Core the apples, but do not cut through the bottom. Peel the
skin one-quarter of the way down from the top of each apple and
place in an 8 x 8 glass baking dish. Pour the apple juice mixture
over the apples and bake for 45 minutes or until the apples are
very tender, basting occasionally.

Soylicious Cheesecake

Serves 8

*Sometimes nothing but the most decadent treat will do.
That doesn't mean it has to be bad for you. Weighing in at under
200 calories per serving, this cheesecake is wonderful for
an occasional guilt-free indulgence.*

Cooking Spray
1/2 cup oat bran
1/2 cup bran cereal, ground
2 teaspoons maple syrup
2 teaspoons trans-fat free soy margarine*
4 10-1/2 ounce boxes of firm reduced-fat silken tofu
3/4 cup sugar
1/2 cup plus 2 tablespoons cashew butter*
1/4 cup cornstarch
Juice and grated peel of 1-1/2 lemons
1 teaspoon vanilla extract
1/2 teaspoon almond extract
Lemon Glaze (recipe follows)

Preheat oven to 400°F. Spray the bottom and sides of an 8-1/2 inch springform pan with cooking spray. Set aside.

Combine the oat bran, cereal, maple syrup and margarine in a small bowl. Using your fingers, mix until crumbly. Press into the bottom of the prepared pan. Bake until golden, approximately 4 to 6 minutes. Cool.

Reduce the oven to 350°F. Combine the tofu, sugar, cashew butter and cornstarch in a food processor. Add the lemon juice, peel and extracts. Blend until smooth, occasionally scraping down the sides of the bowl.

Pour the tofu filling onto the prepared crust and smooth the top using a spatula. Bake until set, approximately 55 to 60 minutes. Turn off the oven and allow the cheesecake to "rest" for 10 minutes.

Remove from oven and set on a wire rack, allowing it to cool completely. Run a knife around the edge of the cake and unhinge the pan. Carefully transfer to a serving plate.

To make the glaze: In a small saucepan, combine 1/2 cup sugar with 1 tablespoon plus 2 teaspoons cornstarch. Using a whisk, gradually add enough water to make a smooth thin paste. Whisk in the juice and grated peel of 2 lemons. Over medium heat, bring the mixture to a boil, stirring constantly.

Remove from the heat and cool completely. Pour over the cheesecake. Chill the finished cheesecake for at least 2 hours before serving. (* Note: Soy margarine and cashew butter are available in most health food stores.)

REMEMBER . . .

➤ Excess weight increases the odds that you'll have a heart attack and that it will occur at a younger age.

➤ Forget fad diets. A well-balanced low-calorie diet that helps you lose one to two pounds a week is the smart way to go.

➤ High salt consumption raises blood pressure.

➤ Not all fats are bad. Essential fatty acids found in some fish, nuts, seeds and vegetable oils are critical for a number of bodily functions.

➤ The saturated fat in meats and dairy products can significantly raise cholesterol levels.

➤ The trans fats in margarine and baked goods have been directly linked to heart disease and high levels increase your risk of a heart attack three-fold.

➤ Adopting the principals of the Mediterranean or Asian diet (which include large amounts of fruits, vegetables and fish) can significantly reduce the risk of developing heart disease.

➤ The antioxidants found in fresh fruits and vegetables help prevent atherosclerosis.

➤ Eating a high-fiber diet naturally lowers LDL cholesterol, homocystine levels and blood pressure.

➤ Soyfoods can tame high cholesterol and are a good source of fiber, the B vitamins and omega-3 fatty acids.

Chapter 5

THE EXERCISE FACTOR

Humans start a natural process of losing muscle and gaining fat at about age 20. This change, though constant, is so gradual that few of us notice it. But if we don't do something to halt and reverse this degenerative process, someday we will find that we can no longer run, go out dancing or even climb a set of stairs.

In a world of remote controls, desk jobs and drive-throughs, far too many of us don't get the exercise we need. Yet, even though a sedentary lifestyle is a well-known risk factor for heart disease, most doctors don't place nearly enough importance on this cost-effective therapy and few give their patients the help they need to implement or stick to a fitness routine.

Exercise plays a powerful and effective role in the prevention and treatment of heart disease. As you'll see in the next section, exercise can significantly boost cardiovascular health and add years to your life.

The Evidence Is In

I'm sure you've seen the ads by fitness gurus featuring trim and beautiful exercise enthusiasts. While it's true that exercise tones your body, it also tones your cardiovascular system. In fact, regular exercise significantly lowers your chances of having a heart attack. And if you've already had one, it can boost your chances of survival. In my book, there is no better medicine than regular exercise.

Study after study has extolled the heart-healthy virtues of exercise. According to the Cooper Institute for Aerobics Research in Dallas, Texas, fit individuals – even those who smoke, have high blood pressure or elevated cholesterol levels –

have a significantly lower death rate than out-of-shape people who don't have *any* of these risk factors.

Imagine, someone who smokes and works out has less chance of dying from heart disease than a smoke-free couch potato! Don't get me wrong – I certainly don't advocate smoking (you'll learn more about this in the next chapter), but it does point out just how powerful exercise is in the fight against heart disease.

Even something as simple as walking can improve your cardiovascular system. According to a large study recently published in the *New England Journal of Medicine*, women (ages 50 to 79) who walked 30 minutes a day, five days a week, reduced their risk of having a heart attack just as much as women who jogged, played tennis or did aerobics for the same amount of time. Both groups cut their risk by a third, regardless of age or weight.

While this and other studies show that you don't need to train like a professional athlete, the length of time spent exercising does matter. After looking at the exercise habits of more than 39,000 women, doctors at Brigham and Women's Hospital concluded that the length of time spent exercising was a much more important factor in reducing heart disease than

Beyond The Heart

Here are some of the additional benefits exercise provides:

- Increases muscle strength
- Boosts energy
- Strengthens bones
- Helps reduce body fat
- Facilitates weight loss
- Improves insulin resistance
- Aids digestion and elimination
- Improves immune function
- Elevates mood
- Reduces stress
- Enhances mental function
- Improves sleep
- Increases self-esteem

the intensity of the workout.

That conclusion was reinforced by researchers at Duke University and East Carolina University, who divided 111 inactive, overweight men and women with poor cholesterol profiles into four exercise groups. After

EXERCISE AND INFLAMMATION

Exercise can also reduce C-reactive protein. Among the nearly 14,000 adults participating in a study by the Centers for Disease Control and Prevention, those who exercised the most had the lowest blood concentrations of CRP.

eight months, all of the participants had a detailed lipoprotein profiling done to see what, if any, changes had occurred as a result of the various exercise programs.

Instead of measuring cholesterol levels, the researchers looked at cholesterol particle size and found that those who exercised the most had the greatest positive changes in the size of their cholesterol particles. (LDL cholesterol is carried by small, dense protein particles, not the larger, fluffy particles that are less likely to clog arteries.) According to the study, the key to developing more large protein particles and decreasing the number of harmful smaller ones – longer stints of exercise.

Even people with more serious heart disease can benefit from exercise. In fact, German physicians at the University of Leipzig Heart Center speculate that physical activity may be even better than surgery for clogged arteries since exercise benefits the whole cardiovascular system while angioplasty opens the arteries only where they are clogged.

To back up their theory, they assigned 73 men with chronic heart failure to either no exercise at all or to two weeks of in-hospital exercise on a stationary bicycle (10 minutes, four to six times a day) followed by six months of exercise for 20 minutes a day at home. By the end of the study, those in the exercise group had significantly better cardiac function, including lower blood pressure, than those in the control group.

Get Moving!

Since aerobic exercise improves cardiovascular fitness and stamina, I've always included it in my workout. Aerobic exercise develops the heart muscle, much the way weight training develops other muscles. The heart grows thicker and stronger while the inside of the heart grows bigger, allowing more blood to be pumped with each heartbeat.

Aerobic activity also improves your blood vessels by increasing nitric oxide, which causes the blood vessels to relax and expand. As we age, blood vessels become stiff, causing our blood pressure to rise. Stiff arteries can also lead to isolated systolic hypertension, a condition that has been linked to an increased risk of stroke and heart disease.

According to a study conducted at the University of Pennsylvania's Institute for Medicine and Engineering, aerobics may increase the flexibility of blood vessels in yet another way. Their research found that, when you exercise, you force more blood through your blood vessels. This elevated blood flow stresses the walls of the vessels as it passes over them, reducing inflammation in a way similar to high doses of steroids.

But the benefits don't stop there. Aerobic exercise offers your heart a number of other positive effects:

√ It improves circulation.

√ It increases the number of capillaries that supply the heart with blood.

√ Your heart rate decreases.

√ LDL levels decrease and HDL levels increase.

Performing aerobics every day will get you in great shape in a hurry. In fact, according to R. James Barnard, Ph.D., professor of physiological science at the University of California, Los Angeles, aerobic activity can significantly improve heart function in less than a month. Dr. Barnard and several of his colleagues took eleven men, who were all about 30 pounds overweight, and let them eat unlimited amounts of whole-wheat bread, pasta, fruit and vegetables. The subjects also exercised for about an hour every day on a treadmill. After just three weeks, the risk factors for the participants had improved dramatically: Oxidative stress had decreased by 28 percent, cholesterol dropped by 19 percent, blood pressure fell by 14 percent, free radicals were cut by 28 percent, and insulin and glucose were reduced by 46 and 70 percent respectively.

Long-term benefits are even more impressive. According to a published report by the University of Texas Southwestern Medical Center, six months of moderate-intensity aerobic exercise can actually make your heart younger. Their study included five middle-aged men who hadn't exercised in years. After participating in a six-month endurance training program, all of the men achieved the aerobic capacity similar to what they had experienced in their 20s!

Your Target Heart Rate

The goal of aerobic exercise is to raise your heart rate to a certain level and keep it there for 20 minutes. When you exercise, your heart beats faster to meet the increased demand for more blood and oxygen. The more intense the activity, the faster your heart will beat. Therefore, keeping an eye on your heart rate during your workout can be an excellent way to monitor exercise intensity.

Figuring out your target heart rate – the optimal rate your heart should beat during aerobic exercise – is a simple, two-step process. First, calculate your maximal heart rate. Then, using that number, you can determine your target heart rate zone.

HEART SMART TIP
GET YOUR CARDIO
When practiced vigorously for a half-hour, these activities are fun and heart-healthy.

Bicycling	Jogging	Spinning classes
Brisk walking	Kick-boxing	Step Aerobics
Circuit weight training	Racquetball	Swimming
Cross-country skiing	Rowing	Synchronized
Swimming or Dancing	Running	Uphill hiking
Elliptical machine workouts	Soccer	Volleyball

Maximal Heart Rate: This number is related to your age, since as you grow older, your heart naturally beats a little more slowly. To estimate your maximal heart rate, simply subtract your age from the number 220.

Target Heart-Rate Zone: This is the number of beats per minute (bpm) at which your heart should be beating during aerobic exercise. For most healthy individuals, this range is 50 to 80 percent of your maximal heart rate. So, if your maximal heart rate is 180 bpm, the low end of the range (50 percent) would be 90 bpm, and the high end of the range (80 percent) would be 144 bpm.

Once you've determined your target heart-rate zone, you need to know how to put that information to good use. These numbers serve as a guideline - an indicator of how hard you should be exercising. Those just beginning an aerobic program should aim for the low end of the zone and pick up the intensity as they become more comfortable with their workout.

Keep in mind that the target heart-rate zone is recommended for individuals without any health problems. Additionally, if you are taking medications that alter the heart rate, consult your doctor before starting an aerobic program.

HEART SMART TIP
Finding Your Pulse

There are a number of "sites" used to monitor the pulse rate. Two convenient sites to use are the radial pulse at the base of the thumb of either hand or the carotid pulse at the side of the neck. By using the first two fingers of one hand and locating the artery, a pulse rate can be easily determined.

Immediately after exercising, isolate your pulse and count the number of beats in a 10-second period. To determine the heart rate in beats per minute, multiply the number of beats per 10 seconds by six. For instance, if your 10-second pulse count is 20, then your heart rate would be 120 bpm.

Walk Away From Heart Disease

Walking is one of the most popular ways to exercise. It's also an excellent way to improve the efficiency of your heart and lose weight. What's more, walking doesn't require any special equipment and carries the least risk of injury of any form of exercise. Best of all, you can do it anywhere, whether you live in the city, the country or somewhere in between.

Several studies have found that brisk walking for three to four hours per week reduces the risk of heart attack and underlying cardiovascular disease in both men and women. For example, researchers working with the Nurse's Health Study estimate that walking at a moderate pace for three or more hours a week reduces a woman's risk of heart attack by about 30 to 40 percent. Similar results have been found in studies of men.

The hours spent walking can increase HDL levels, even when the intensity isn't high enough to cause much improvement in cardiovascular fitness. Walking on a regular basis is also ideal for people who are trying to bring their blood pressure under control.

HEART SMART TIP

Although walking is something you've done all your life, there are a few things to keep in mind before you begin:

- Find a pair of comfortable walking shoes — nothing undermines your daily walk faster then a painful blister or two.

- Walk briskly and practice good posture. Develop a good breathing pattern and keep your body aligned and relaxed.

- Walk everyday. If inclement weather threatens your plans, try doing a few laps through a shopping mall or use a treadmill if you have access to one.

If you're not used to exercising, start slowly, limiting yourself to a 10 minute walk. As your stamina increases, you should be able to increase your walk to 45 minutes.

Win With Weight Training

As wonderful as aerobic exercise is for the heart, it should be balanced by resistance training, more commonly known as weight lifting. Resistance training improves the muscles and nerve pathways that direct and control movement. It also increases strength and general fitness, including enhanced function of the respiratory, cardiac and metabolic systems.

For years, the cardiovascular benefits of resistance training were thought to be merely a side effect of lifting weights. But over the last decade, it has become clear that weight-training decreases heart rate, reduces blood pressure, improves cholesterol profiles, fortifies artery flexibility and increases cardiorespiratory fitness.

Here's another bonus: Resistance training thickens muscles – and the more muscle you have, the more calories you will burn.

Like aerobics, resistance training burns calories during the workout. The difference is that, once you're finished doing your aerobics, your body quickly stops burning calories. But after you've finished a weight lifting routine, your body continues burning calories for up to one hour.

Along with elevating your metabolic rate and strengthening your muscles, weight lifting also increases your bone density. And increased bone density is a frontline defense in the war against the bone thinning disease, osteoporosis.

> **HEART SMART TIP**
>
> To prevent sore muscles and possible injury, it's wise to start slowly. Choose the lowest weight possible and start by doing 10 to 12 on each side. Over the next few weeks, increase the weight and the number of repetitions.

Many health clubs, colleges and recreation centers are equipped with both free weights and weight machines. But before you begin, make sure you get instruction on the proper way to use the equipment. Although committing to a regular weight training routine - at least three times a week - may require a bit of will-power, you'll be rewarded with a stronger, leaner body and a healthier heart.

Stretch The Benefits

Years ago, stretching served as an introduction to exercise. The thought was that warming up cold muscles before heavy exercise kept them from becoming injured. But now, most fitness experts have realized that stretching cold muscles can actually cause injury.

Think of it this way: If you put a rubber band in the freezer and then stretch it, it snaps. It's the same idea with muscles and connective tissue.   Instead of stretching before you work out, try jogging in place for a few minutes to increase the blood flow to your muscles so that they are more easily extended. Save the heavy-duty stretching for after your workout.

Stretching keeps the muscles and connective tissues supple, improves posture and helps keep you flexible. While you should stretch every part of your body, pay a little more attention to chronically tight

Safety Alert!
Avoid these stretching mistakes
- Don't bounce. Holding a stretch is more effective and there is less risk of injury.
- Don't stretch a "cold" muscle.
- If a stretch hurts, ease up.
- Don't hold your breath.

muscles. But if you experience any pain during a stretch, you're either going too far or you may have strained a muscle during your workout.

Stretches should be performed slowly and smoothly. If you are a novice, begin gently with simple stretches and hold each stretch for a minimum of 10 to 30 seconds. As your flexibility begins to improve, you should be able to accomplish more complex stretches for longer periods of time.

The East-West Connection

Incorporating Eastern culture into Western exercise is the latest trend in fitness – and one that I wholeheartedly support. Activities like yoga, tai chi and qi gong are a wonderful way for both sedentary people and exercise enthusiasts to get in shape. Best of all, these forms of exercise don't require any special equipment and can be practiced by anyone, regardless of age.

Yoga originated as a spiritual practice over six thousand years ago. Over the past thirty years, however, the western world has adopted yoga as a therapeutic form of exercise that emphasizes deep breathing, relaxed movements and mental concentration. Among its many benefits, yoga enhances flexibility, increases strength and improves circulation. It also cultivates balance and reduces stress.

Yoga is simply a series of "asanas" or poses which are best learned and practiced under the guidance of a qualified teacher. Although there are a number of well-illustrated and comprehensive books on the subject, it's a difficult art to master from a series of pictures. Fortunately, a number of yoga centers have established themselves across the country and offer enjoyable classes suited to all levels of mastery, from beginner to advanced. In addition, classes can often be found through your local community center or college.

Although *T'ai Chi* is a centuries-old offshoot of yoga, it departs from the still-life asanas of yoga into the world of moving meditation. The heart of the practice is the Chinese concept of "chi," roughly translated to mean the life force or vital energy of the universe. This energy flows through all of nature, including human beings.

Based on the movements of animals, t'ai chi is composed of slow dance-like steps and gestures. The weight of the body shifts continually from one foot to the other as the movements are performed in a series of circles, arcs and spirals. The fluidity and grace of this form of exercise encourages relaxation and mental peace, as well as balance and flexibility. A qualified instructor is essential and classes are offered at many martial arts schools and health clubs.

Qigong is an ancient Taoist system of exercise which compliments both yoga and t'ai chi. Healing qigong combines breathwork, gentle movements and meditative postures to harmonize the body, mind and spirit. Because of its positive effect on strength, stamina, flexibility, posture and concentration, the practice of qigong will enhance your physical performance, improve sleep, help balance stress, boost energy levels, and clarify your mind. Unfortunately, there aren't many qigong classes available at this time, but it is easy to learn and there are some excellent videos on the market.

How Much Is Enough?

The Institute of Medicine recently released new guidelines calling for one hour of daily physical activity – up from the 30-minute goal touted by many other health organizations. But that doesn't mean you have to do one hour of sustained activity a day. Break it up into more manageable and more enjoyable segments. If you work out for 30 minutes in the morning, take a half-hour walk in the afternoon. Or play some golf or tennis. Not only will this routine keep your cardiovascular system in shape, it will also keep your weight down and your muscles toned.

But if you're new to exercise or very out-of-shape, start slowly – try five minutes on an exercise bike followed by 10 minutes of resistance training. Then increase the time you spend on each activity by a few minutes each day until you are getting an hour of activity every day.

Stick To It

Starting an exercise program is fairly easy. Sticking with it year in and year out is quite another matter. Every January, gyms and health clubs are filled with enthusiastic exercisers. But by April, many of these folks are nowhere to be seen.

The goal, of course, is to make exercise a regular and enjoyable part of your daily life. Here are a few motivational tips to help keep you moving:

√ Find activities you enjoy. After all, if you don't like exercising, you won't do it.

√ Get an exercise buddy. Surrounding yourself with supportive people will keep you going.

√ Join an exercise class. Just signing up for a class forces you to schedule it into your routine.

√ Try a trainer. Professional trainers can help you remember why you started exercising in the first place.

√ Set exercise goals. Tap into your competitive nature and see how long it takes to achieve your goals.

√ Keep a record of your activities. Reward yourself at special milestones.

√ Vary your routine. Doing the same thing every day becomes monotonous. Continually look for new ways to enjoy working out.

REMEMBER ...

➤ People who exercise live longer.

➤ It's not how hard you work out that counts, but how long.

➤ Regular exercise reduces cholesterol, blood pressure and CRP.

➤ Aerobic exercise strengthens the heart and improves blood vessel health.

➤ Other benefits of a cardiovascular workout include a lower heart rate, less free radical damage and an increase in capillaries.

➤ For the most benefit, sustain your target heart rate for at least 20 minutes.

➤ Walking is an excellent aerobic activity.

➤ Balance your aerobic exercise with weight training. Lifting weights not only strengthens muscles, it decreases heart rate and blood pressure, improves your cholesterol profile and boosts artery flexibility.

➤ Don't stretch before your workout. Wait until after to perform deep stretching.

➤ Explore more exotic forms of exercise like yoga or tai chi.

➤ Make exercise fun!

Chapter 6

LIFESTYLE CHOICES FOR
A HEALTHY HEART

Along with diet and exercise, there are other things you can do to lower your risk of heart disease. Four areas that deserve special consideration are sleep, smoking, stress and, odd as it may sound, your dental health. Anyone concerned with heart disease needs to pay special attention to all of these risk factors.

Reigning in these potential problems will not only benefit your heart, it will set you on a path toward optimum health. Fortunately, because heart disease develops over a long period of time, we have many opportunities throughout our lives to make positive changes.

HEART SMART TIP
Beating Insomnia

- Set a regular bedtime.
- Try a warm bath.
- Make sure the room is dark and quiet.
- Take supplemental calcium or melatonin 30 minutes before bedtime.
- Herbs like valerian or passion-flower can also induce sleep.

Sleep

When was the last time you got a good night's sleep? As the pace of life seems to quicken with each passing year, it can be difficult to log your eight hours. But chronic sleep deprivation can increase your risk of heart disease.

As part of the Nurse's Health Study, researchers at Vancouver General Hospital set out to discover what, if any, impact sleep had on the risk of developing coronary heart disease. More than 71,000 women without heart disease were asked about their sleep habits. A decade later the group had recorded a total of 934 heart attacks, including 271 fatal attacks. After analyzing the data, the Vancouver team found that the women who reported sleeping five hours

HEART SMART TIP

Since being overweight can trigger sleep apnea, some people find relief by losing just 10 percent of their weight.

or less were 45 percent more likely to develop heart disease than women who slept eight hours a night. On the flip side, the researchers found that women who routinely slept nine hours or more a night also had a higher risk.

But it isn't just the time you put in sleeping that can adversely affect your cardiovascular system. When it comes to heart disease, quality also counts. Snoring may signal that you have obstructive sleep apnea, a condition that causes the throat to close and results in short interruptions in your breathing. According to a Mayo Clinic study, sleep apnea raises blood pressure, lowers blood oxygen levels and stretches the walls of the atria, making them susceptible to irregular electrical rhythms – a condition called atrial fibrillation.

Atrial fibrillation is the most common heart arrhythmia. But, as common as it may be, it can have serious consequences. When the upper chambers of the heart quiver rapidly and erratically – as many as 400 times a minute – blood does not move efficiently through the heart. This pooling blood is more likely to clot, leading to heart attacks or strokes. The condition can also lead to heart failure by causing the heart's main pumping chambers, the ventricles, to contract rapidly – often more than 100 beats per minute.

Although serious cases of sleep apnea may require surgery, the most common treatment is nasal *continuous positive airway pressure* (CPAP). The patient wears a mask over the nose while they sleep, and pressure from an air blower forces air through the nasal passages. The air pressure is adjusted so that it is just

Safety Alert!

Here are some facts that should make every smoker think twice before they light up:

- Smoking lowers HDL cholesterol.
- Smoking deteriorates the elastic properties of the aorta, the largest blood vessel in the body, which increases the risk for developing blood clots.
- Smoking increases the activity of the sympathetic nervous system, putting additional stress on the system that regulates the heart and blood vessels.
- Smokers have twice the risk of having a heart attack than non-smokers.
- Smokers who have a heart attack are more likely to die, and die suddenly, than non-smokers.
- Those who smoke a pack of cigarettes a day have almost two and a half times the risk for having a stroke as nonsmokers.
- People exposed to second-hand smoke have a 30 percent higher risk of developing heart disease.

enough to prevent the throat from collapsing during sleep.

Smoking

Let's face it, every smoker knows that cigarettes are bad for their health, yet millions of people smoke anyway. If you are one of them and have or are at risk for heart disease, quitting is one of the very best things you can do for your heart.

I know that quitting is much easier said than done. Over the past 20 years, I've taught smoking cessation to many of my patients and one thing is clear – cigarettes are more addictive than either heroin or cocaine. And it isn't just the nicotine that keeps you coming back for more. There is evidence that other chemical components in cigarettes can also cause a physical and psychological dependence. But, while smoking is the most difficult habit to change, it can be done.

Fortunately, there are a number of ways to quit – nicotine patches, acupuncture, hypnosis, even drugs. Personally, I've found that a combination approach works best for many of my patients and so my program incorporates behavior modification, acupuncture, nicotine patches or gum, and hypnotherapy. The results have truly been amazing, with up to a 98% success rate.

No matter what it takes, quitting can greatly benefit your health. Consider this: Smoking will significantly in-crease your risk of heart disease. The more you smoke, and the longer you have smoked, the greater the risk. Even light smokers, who may smoke only 1-14 cigarettes a day, have a three times greater risk of developing heart disease than non-smokers.

HEART SMART TIP
What Happens When You Quit Smoking

➤ Within 30 minutes of quitting smoking, your pulse rate slows down and blood pressure drops toward normal.

➤ Within hours of stopping, the level of carbon monoxide in your blood drops, enabling the blood to carry more oxygen.

➤ Two days after quitting, nerve endings begin to recover and your sense of smell and taste begin to return.

➤ Within 72 hours of quitting, lung volume increases.

➤ Months after quitting, shortness of breath diminishes.

➤ In the first year, the risk of heart attack attributed to smoking declines for both men and women.

➤ After 10 years, the risk of developing cancer is about the same as for nonsmokers.

Source: www.quitsmoking.com

Of the 4,000 or so chemicals identified in cigarette smoke, the most damaging to the cardiovascular system are nicotine and carbon monoxide. Nicotine causes an immediate increase in blood pressure, heart rate, cardiac output and coronary blood flow. Carbon monoxide binds to hemoglobin, which reduces the amount of oxygen delivered to tissues. There is also evidence that smoking repeatedly damages the lining of blood vessels, setting a smoker up for atherosclerosis.

If you don't succeed the first time you try to quit, don't give up. Studies show that smokers who have tried smoking cessation in the past have a much better chance of staying smoke-free with each successive attempt. However you choose to stop, just do it! This is one risk factor that is simply not negotiable.

Stress

Stress has been with us since the beginning of time. That's not necessarily bad. Short-term stress can generate the impetus necessary to convert thought into action, whether that action is planting a garden, meeting a deadline or escaping from a fire. But when stress becomes a routine part of our lives, it can spell trouble – especially if we don't learn how to manage it. More than 70 percent of all doctor visits are because of stress-related disease, many of which involved the heart. In fact, people who live in a high state of anxiety are 4.5 times more likely to die of a heart attack or stroke.

The primary reason that long-term stress can have

> ### Safety Alert!
>
> Even short bouts of stress can lead to heart damage, say researchers at Ohio State University.
>
> In their study of 35 women, they discovered that stress slows the body's ability to clear triglycerides from the blood. And the longer these unhealthy fats circulate in your body, the more negative impact they have on your heart.

such deadly consequences is that it triggers a hormone called cortisol. In a study of 18 healthy male doctors, researchers at the Humboldt University of Berlin, Germany, found that high cortisol levels can cause red blood cells to clump together. The blood becomes thick and sluggish, increasing the risk of hypertension, stroke and heart attack. Over time, stress can also change artery walls, causing them to become ridged.

According to recent evidence, living the anxious life can also have a negative impact on your lipids. University of Pittsburg researchers conducted a clinical study of 688 middle-aged women suffering from recurrent chest pain and found that those prone to high levels of stress and anger had a more than four-fold greater risk of high LDL.

But here's the good news: A growing number of studies suggest that stress management can help reduce the detrimental effects of stress on your heart. One study in the journal *Archives of Internal Medicine* found that people with severe hypertension were able to significantly reduce their blood pressure after ten hours of stress management therapy.

A Duke University study of 94 men with heart disease also found that those who learned relaxation techniques had fewer heart attacks, less cardiac surgery and lower medical costs than those who didn't learn how to manage their stress. So do yourself and your heart a favor. Try one of the following techniques to help you get a handle on stress.

Biofeedback: Biofeedback is a treatment technique in which people are trained to improve their health by using signals from their own bodies. Using monitoring equipment, biofeedback is often aimed at changing habitual reactions to stress that can cause disease. Many clinicians believe that some patients have forgotten how to relax.

Feedback of physical responses such as skin temperature and muscle tension provides information to help patients recognize a relaxed state. If you think you might benefit from biofeedback therapy, look for a biofeedback therapist that will assist you in treating your hypertension and other stress-related disorders. To locate a biofeedback therapist in your area, check the resources at the end of this book.

Meditation: There are several different types of meditation, including

Safety Alert!

Biofeedback is very safe. However, if you are undergoing any sort of medical treatment, you should consult your doctor before beginning therapy.

Biofeedback should not be used as a substitute for proper medical attention since it may mask the symptoms of a more serious condition.

mindfulness meditation, concentrative meditation and transcendental meditation (TM). Of those, TM is perhaps the most widely studied. Not only does TM induce mental relaxation, studies show that this form of meditation reduces the risk of hypertension, angina and atherosclerosis. One reason for this, say researchers at Reina Sofia Hospital in Cordoba, Spain, is that the regular practice of TM has a significant effect on the sympathetic nervous system. In their study, 19 practitioners of TM were compared with 16 volunteers who had never used any type of relaxation therapy. Throughout the study, the researchers measured the amounts of norepinephrine and epinephrine in the participant's blood and found that those practicing TM had consistently lower plasma levels of these stress hormones.

Another study, recently presented at a meeting of the American Heart Association, found that TM reduced the severity of risk factors in Syndrome X. The researchers noted that the people who meditated decreased their blood pressure, blood sugar and insulin. Other research has found that meditation helps the body and mind so much that some patients can reduce their medications, especially drugs used to treat hypertension and anxiety.

No matter what type of meditation you choose, each form requires daily practice and I advise learning from a master. The investment you make learning to meditate will more than pay for itself in improved health and well-being.

HEART SMART TIP

2-Minute Relaxation

Find a quiet corner where you won't be disturbed. Take a couple of deep breaths and let your body flop for a minute or two. Slowly come up into an erect position.

Practicing this exercise each day has a cumulative effect on your stress levels and will prevent them from escalating.

Muscle Relaxation: This method of stress control involves contracting and relaxing the large muscle groups in your body until each part of your body is free from tension. This form of relaxation doesn't require any special equipment or training. Simply lie on your back, arms at your sides, and begin to breathe deeply. Tense each muscle group, starting with your feet, for a count of 10 and then relax. Move to the next muscle group and repeat, remembering to breathe. End by tightening and relaxing the muscles in your face. Then take a few more deep, even breaths before slowly getting up.

Relax With Music: One of the easiest ways to reduce stress is by simply listening to some soothing music. In a study of recent heart attack victims, those who listened to music for twenty-minutes experienced a reduction in respiration and heart rate, as

Safety Alert!

When listening to music through headphones, take care to keep the music at a low volume. Prolonged playing of loud music can cause permanent hearing damage.

well as a drop in oxygen demands by the heart. Anxiety was also reduced, an effect that lasted for 30 minutes after the music stopped.

Music therapy is an ideal do-it-yourself way to combat stress. Although special therapeutic tapes and CDs are readily available through either mail-order or from specialty bookstores, they may not suit your musical tastes. Instead, choose some soothing music from your own collection. This type of stress-reduction works best if you are relaxed and comfortable, and are able to fully concentrate on the music.

Stress-Busting Herbs: Herbs have been used for centuries to calm anxiety, counteract insomnia and help people adapt to stressful situations. Nervines, like kava kava or passionflower, can soothe mild to moderate anxiety without the adverse side effects common to many of the drugs often prescribed for anxiety. Adaptogenic herbs, which include ginseng and rhodiola, can also help your body resist the negative effects of stress. Numerous studies have found that both of these herbs also enhance concentration and promote overall well-being.

See Your Dentist

Most of us don't make the connection between good dental care and heart disease. But some new studies have found that patients with gum disease and tooth decay are at an increased risk for heart disease.

In one study, Dr. Pirkko J. Pussinen, from the University of Helsinki, and

Safety Alert!

If you have heart disease, make sure to let your dentist know – especially if you are taking Coumadin. This drug can cause excessive bleeding during extractions or root canals unless proper precautions are taken.

For patients with heart murmurs or replacement heart valves, antibiotics will be needed before, during and shortly after conventional dental treatments.

colleagues looked for antibodies to two common types of dental bacteria in the blood of 1,163 men. Antibodies are chemicals produced by the body to fight infection and are an indirect way of determining whether a particular bug is present. Men with antibodies to the dental bacteria were 50 percent more likely to have heart disease than men without these antibodies. Gum disease has also been linked to higher LDL and total cholesterol. The lesson here is that brushing and flossing are important, not only for your smile, but for your heart. And regular visits to your dentist are essential.

REMEMBER . . .

➤ You need eight hours of sleep every night. Too little or too much can increase the risk of heart disease.

➤ Snoring may be a sign of a sleep disorder that can lead to a heart attack or stroke.

➤ Smoking is the absolute worst thing for your heart. It substantially increases ALL cardiovascular risk factors.

➤ If you don't smoke, don't start. If you do, quit now!

➤ People under constant stress are 4.5 times more likely to die of a heart attack or stroke.

➤ Stress not only causes red blood cells to become thick and sluggish, it can also cause artery walls to become ridged.

➤ Even short-term stress can damage the heart since it reduces the body's ability to clear triglycerides.

➤ Practiced regularly, stress-reduction techniques can reduce blood pressure and heart rate. It can also improve your cholesterol profile.

➤ Stress reduction can be as complex as biofeedback or as simple as listening to music. Choose a technique (or combination of techniques) that fit your schedule and comfort level.

➤ Gingivitis (gum disease) and tooth decay increase the risk of heart disease. Make sure to visit your dentist regularly.

Chapter 7

DIETARY SUPPLEMENTS FOR HEART HEALTH

When it comes to preventing or reversing heart disease, nothing can take the place of a low-fat diet based on fresh fruits, vegetables and whole grains. But, since diet alone often isn't enough, you may need to add supplements.

Most of these natural supplements are considered safe when taken at the recommended doses. However, if you are considering adding supplements at doses higher than the recommendations I've made below, it's a good idea to consult a professional before you begin.

If you have a pre-existing medical condition – and especially if you have suffered a heart attack – you should *always* talk to your doctor before taking supplements of any kind. Although dietary supplements normally have fewer side effects than prescription drugs, some can interact with your medications, enhancing or decreasing the effect of your prescription.

Finally, like most things in life, quality counts. When shopping for supplements, choose natural over synthetic whenever possible. Natural supplements are often more potent and easier for the body to use.

Vitamins

According to conventional nutritionists, if you eat a balanced diet that contains six to 10 servings of fruits and vegetables, you're getting all of the

---

HEART SMART TIP
Maximize Your Multi

When shopping for a multivitamin, look for one that also includes a variety of heart-healthy minerals, including calcium, magnesium and selenium. And check the label for other nutrients like antioxidants, green foods and herbs that support cardiovascular health.

---

vitamins you need. HOGWASH! Because of modern farming practices and food processing, many of the nutrients in our fruits and vegetables have been depleted. In other words, our food just isn't as nutritious as it used to be.

Did You Know?

This potent antioxidant can help lower CRP. According to a new study by researchers at Tufts University, consuming 250 mg. of vitamin C twice a day can effectively lower plasma CRP levels in both men and women.

One way to correct this lack of natural nutrition is by taking a multivitamin every day. In fact, the American Medical Association even advises a daily multivitamin for all Americans. But most over-the-counter multivitamins contain only a smidgen of the essential vitamins we need. The recommended daily allowances (RDAs) or "daily values" listed on vitamin labels are only the amounts the average adult needs to prevent a deficiency – not the amounts required to achieve your best health. They certainly aren't the levels needed to prevent or reverse heart disease.

That said, a multivitamin can provide you with some insurance against disease. But the following vitamins can be added as needed to give you even more protection.

Vitamin C: This free radical fighter plays an extremely important role in heart health. But, unlike animals, the human body can't manufacture its own supply. And, because vitamin C is water-soluble, the body can't store it, so it must be replenished every day.

In one famous study conducted at the University of California, Los Angeles,

How Much Should I Take?

Since fewer than one in ten people eat the recommended daily servings of fruits and vegetables, I recommend taking 1,000 to 2,000 mg. of vitamin C a day.

researchers analyzed the vitamin C intake of more than 11,000 people over 10 years. They found that men who consumed more than 300 mg. of vitamin C a day had a 45 percent lower risk of dying from heart disease than men who only got 50 mg. or less a day. And, while women didn't fare quite as well, vitamin C also cut their risk by 25 percent.

Another recent study involving 11,349 adults found that vitamin C had a statistically significant benefit in preventing heart disease, and some researchers have noted that low levels are associated with an increase in heart attacks.

Although vitamin C is most often thought of as an immune booster, it protects against atherosclerosis. Not only does it inhibit platelet aggregation, this potent antioxidant plays a role in protecting LDL cholesterol from oxidation. Vitamin C is also crucial for the production of collagen, an important protein that helps to maintain the integrity of blood vessels and other tissues.

If that weren't enough, vitamin C decreases the level of those proteins that contribute to blood clots. Other activities of this crucial antioxidant include lowering lipoprotein(a), elevating HDL cholesterol and regenerating vitamin E.

Vitamin E: Vitamin E is one of the most commonly used vitamins. In fact, more doctors add this potent antioxidant to their health care routine than any other supplement. No wonder – the Health Professional's Follow-Up Study of 39,910 men found that those who took the most vitamin E had a 40 percent lower risk of heart disease.

Vitamin E may also prevent heart attacks in

How Much Should I Take?

I advise all of my patients to take 400 to 800 IU of vitamin E a day. Vitamin E supplements are so safe that the National Academy of Sciences has established the daily tolerable upper intake level for adults to be 1,000 mg of vitamin E.

HEART SMART TIP

Shopping for vitamin E can be confusing. The vitamin E you'll find in drug and health food stores is usually preceded by either a "d" or "dl," depending on its chemical structure. While "d-alpha tocopherol" means you are getting a natural, more active form of vitamin E, "dl-tocopherol" refers to a synthetic compound.

According to chemists specializing in this fat-soluble vitamin, the natural form may be as much as twice as bioavailable as synthetic vitamin E. And vitamin E supplements that are labeled as "mixed tocopherols" may be the most beneficial since they contain not only alpha-tocopherol, but also beta-, gamma- and delta-tocopherols.

people who already have atherosclerosis. The Cambridge Heart Antioxidant Study (CHAOS) tested the effects of vitamin E on future cardiovascular events in patients with atherosclerosis. The results were impressive – vitamin E reduced the risk of a subsequent heart attack by 77 percent and the risk of all cardiovascular events by 47 percent.

Scientists are also discovering that vitamin E lowers CRP levels. Researchers at the University of Texas Southwestern Medical Center gave 1,200 IU of vitamin E to diabetic patients with high CRP levels every day for three months. By the end of the trial, the Texas team found a significant decrease in CRP and suggested that vitamin E could be an effective therapy in the prevention of atherosclerosis.

B-Complex Vitamins: Like antioxidants, the B vitamins appear to work together, particularly when it comes to lowering homocystine. And three of these B vitamins appear to be superstars:

√ **Folic acid** effectively lowers homocystine levels and decreases inflammation. In fact, studies have shown that folic acid alone can cut homocystine levels by 50 percent. But don't expect this to happen at the 400 mcg. usually recommended. You need to take 800 to 1,000 mcg. a day to effectively battle high homocystine levels.

√ **Vitamin B-6** is another heart protector that inhibits the formation of homocystine and aids in the prevention of arteriosclerosis. It also helps the body absorb vitamin B-12 and magnesium. Vitamin B-6 is usually considered safe up to 200 mg. a day. More than that can damage sensory nerves, leading to numbness in the hands and feet as well as difficulty walking.

√ **Vitamin B-12:** This B vitamin also helps lower homocystine and aids folic acid in regulating the formation of red blood cells. The recommended dose is 500 to 1,000 mcg. in a sublingual form (which is dissolved under the tongue) to insure better absorption.

Another one of the B vitamins, niacin, has been used for years to lower cholesterol. In one clinical trial, researchers compared niacin to a popular statin drug. One-hundred and thirty-six people with high cholesterol were randomly assigned to receive either niacin or lovastatin. While both groups saw benefits, the statin was slightly more effective at lowering LDL cholesterol. But, when it came to HDL, those in the niacin group experienced a 33 percent increase compared to only seven percent for the statin group.

But niacin can be tricky. One controlled study has found that 1,000 mg. of niacin per day or more raised homocystine levels. This B

How Much Should I Take?

To prevent heart disease, look for a vitamin B complex that contains 400 mcg. of folic acid, at least 50 mg. of vitamin B-6 and 500 to 1,000 mcg. of B-12.

vitamin can also cause flushing and is not tolerated well by some people. If you are considering taking niacin to lower your cholesterol, look for non-flushing niacin or take one baby aspirin with your niacin to prevent flushing.

Beta-Carotene: This precursor to vitamin A is one of the carotenoids – plant pigments that act like powerful antioxidants. One clinical trial of 1,400 people throughout Europe found that those with the highest levels of beta-carotene in their bloodstream had the lowest risk of suffering from a heart attack.

How Much Should I Take?

The most common beta-carotene dosage is 25,000 IU a day, though some people take considerably more than this. Unlike vitamin A, beta carotene isn't toxic at high doses.

Of course, dietary sources of this antioxidant are best and can be found in dark green and orange or yellow vegetables. But if you aren't eating enough vegetables, it's a good idea to supplement with this important vitamin precursor.

Lycopene: Most of us are familiar with lycopene as a nutrient that promotes prostate health. But this carotenoid (which is found in tomatoes, watermelon and pink grapefruit) has recently been targeted by researchers for its ability to protect against heart disease.

How Much Should I Take?

Although no specific recommendations have been established for lycopene, it's wise to choose a multivitamin that includes this potent antioxidant.

In the most recent study, researchers at Brigham and Women's Hospital and Harvard Medical School followed more than 28,000 middle-aged and elderly disease-free women for more than four years. By the end of the study, the joint team of researchers found that the women with the highest lycopene levels had a 50 percent lower risk of developing heart disease than those with the lowest levels.

These findings add to a growing body of research linking lycopene levels to cardiovascular disease. For example, the European Study of Antioxidants, Myocardial Infarction and Cancer of the Breast (EURAMIC) studied adipose tissue for lycopene concentration and risk for cardiovascular disease. That study found that men with the highest levels of lycopene in their adipose tissue were 48 percent less likely to develop cardiovascular disease. The Kuopio Ischaemic Heart Disease Risk Factor Study also found that low serum lycopene levels were associated with increased risk of heart attack and stroke.

One reason lycopene has such a critical impact on heart disease is because it helps prevent the oxidation of LDL cholesterol. University of Toronto investigators found that consuming one to two servings per day of tomato juice, spaghetti sauce and supplemental lycopene for just one week doubled blood levels of lycopene, while notably lowering oxidized LDL levels. Preliminary research has also linked low lycopene levels in the blood to higher CRP levels.

Minerals

As important as vitamins are, they can't be assimilated without the aid of minerals. And though the body can manufacture a few vitamins, it can't manufacture a single mineral.

All of the tissues and internal fluids in our bodies contain varying quantities of minerals, including soft tissue, muscle and blood. While they are vital to overall mental and physical well-being, certain minerals, like the ones listed below, are particularly important to cardiovascular health.

Calcium: Known as the bone-building mineral, calcium also plays a role in heart health. In one cohort study, researchers at the

University of South Carolina analyzed data from more than 34,000 postmenopausal women found that those taking the most calcium for bone health also had a significantly lower risk of atherosclerosis.

While this important mineral appears to lower LDL cholesterol by slowing down the amount of saturated fat that is absorbed into the bloodstream, women taking calcium supplements may also have higher HDL cholesterol. In one clinical trial, 223 postmenopausal women were randomly assigned to take a placebo or 1,000 mg. of calcium each day for one year. At the beginning and the end of the intervention, researchers measured the blood levels of the participants' total cholesterol, as well as LDL and HDL cholesterol.

After a year of taking calcium, the researchers noted a slight reduction in LDL cholesterol. But HDL levels increased by 7 percent compared to the levels before supplementation. And HDL levels increased significantly more in the women taking calcium than in those taking the placebo.

Population-based studies have also suggested a link between calcium deficiency and high blood pressure. One study monitored elderly patients with hypertension for 24 hours to evaluate the effect of calcium supplementation on blood pressure. After taking 1,000 mg. of elemental calcium, systolic and diastolic blood pressure declined by 13.6 mmHg and 5.0 mmHg

How Much Should I Take?

While dairy products, salmon and dark-green vegetables are all good sources of calcium, it's hard to get adequate amounts of this important mineral through diet alone, so it's wise to take 1,000 to 1,500 mg. of supplemental calcium a day. But be aware that the body can't absorb more than 500 mg. of calcium at a time, so take your supplements in divided doses.

respectively. Other research has found that taking supplemental calcium also helps to maintain the flexibility of blood vessel walls.

Magnesium: Without this essential mineral, your heart would cease to function properly. In fact, when researchers from the University of Virginia examined the dietary magnesium intake in 7,172 men who took part in the Honolulu Heart Program, they found that the rate of heart disease was significantly lower in those with the highest daily magnesium intake (340 mg. or more) compared with those with the lowest intake (186 mg. or less).

No wonder – magnesium increases the heart's supply of oxygen, lowers cholesterol, hinders blood vessel blockages and prevents the formation of blood clots. It also relaxes the smooth muscles in the arteries and can restore normal rhythm.

Additionally, population-based research has found that people with high serum levels of magnesium have lower blood pressure. In one crossover trial, 60 hypertensive people were assigned to take either a magnesium supplement or a placebo for eight weeks. The two groups then traded places – those on magnesium were switched to the placebo and vice versa. By the end of the study, blood pressure was significantly lower during the time the patients were taking magnesium – and the best results were seen in those with the highest blood pressure at the beginning of the study.

Magnesium has also been called "nature's calcium channel blocker" because it prevents calcium from entering cells. The

> ### How Much Should I Take?
>
> Because magnesium enhances the absorption of calcium, both supplements should be taken together. The recommended dose is 500 to 750 mg. a day, balanced in a 1:2 ratio with calcium.

result is that the artery walls relax, allowing more blood to flow through them. Yet magnesium has none of the adverse side effects common to pharmaceutical channel blockers.

Selenium: This trace mineral plays an important role in the oxidation of lipids and low levels have been linked to atherosclerosis. In one investigation, researchers tested 55 men and 71 women living in a rural Japanese seaside village and found that those with a moderate to high selenium intake also had elevated HDL levels – leading the investigators to conclude that selenium is an important factor in the prevention of heart disease.

While selenium is naturally found in the soil, it is severely depleted in the U.S. As a result, the foods we eat often don't contain sufficient amounts of this mineral to meet our requirements.

Antioxidants

As I discussed in Chapter 4, free radicals are unstable molecules that can damage the arteries and oxidize LDL cholesterol (which contributes to plaque build-up). But nature has an ingenious weapon against oxidation – antioxidants.

How Much Should I Take?

You only need about 200 mcg. a day and your daily multivitamin should contain this much. But don't take more than this amount, since toxicity is possible and may harm the thyroid and nervous system.

Antioxidants block the process of oxidation by neutralizing free radicals. In other words, they convert free radicals to harmless waste products that get eliminated from your body before they can do damage. But in doing so, the antioxidants themselves become oxidized. That is why there is a constant need to replenish our antioxidant resources.

Along with vitamins C, E, beta carotene and selenium, the antioxidants that follow play a special role in heart health.

Alpha Lipoic Acid: Although not a true vitamin, alpha lipoic acid (ALA) is a vitamin-like antioxidant that is soluble in both fat and water. One of its most valuable qualities is that it can re-activate other heart-healthy antioxidants, including vitamin C, vitamin E and coenzyme-Q10.

New evidence out of Canada shows that ALA can modulate blood lipids, protect against LDL oxidation and help lower blood pressure. ALA also improves a number of functions in the heart including oxygen uptake, cardiac output and energy production. Not only does ALA act like an antioxidant itself, it also stimulates the production of glutathione, giving cells a double dose of antioxidants.

How Much Should I Take?

Although the best source of ALA is through foods like spinach, beef liver and yeast, most of us don't eat these foods on a regular basis. For general antioxidant protection, I recommend supplementing your diet with 100 mg. of ALA twice a day.

This antioxidant is easily absorbed when taken orally, and once inside the cells, it is quickly converted to its most potent form, dihydrolipoic acid. Because both ALA acid and dihydrolipoic acid are antioxidants, their combined actions give them greater antioxidant potency than any natural antioxidant now known.

Coenzyme Q-10: Co-Q10 plays an important role in providing energy to the cells, especially those in the heart, and low levels are implicated in virtually all cardiovascular diseases, including angina, hypertension, cardiomyopathy and congestive heart failure. Unfortunately, Co-Q10 levels decrease as we get older. And, statin drugs deplete stores of this critical nutrient, making it an indispensable supplement for anyone taking these medications.

While this enzyme is a potent anti-inflammatory, Co-Q10's

most important role in heart disease is its ability to lower blood pressure by decreasing oxidative stress and insulin response. Co-Q10 also has a positive effect on lipoproteins and HDL cholesterol.

A few years ago, the *International Journal of Cardiology* published the results of a double-blind trial which tested the effects of Co-Q10 on 47 patients who had either suffered a heart

> ## How Much Should I Take?
>
> Co-Q10 is present in a number of foods, including beef, poultry and broccoli. But if you have heart disease, Co-Q10 should be high on your list of essential supplements. I recommend taking a minimum of 60 mg. of Co-Q10 twice a day, preferably with meals to ensure its absorption. Double the dose (120 mg.) if you're taking statin drugs.

attack or had been diagnosed with angina. Twenty-five of the patients received 60 mg. of Co-Q10 a day, while everyone else got a placebo. In less than a month, those on the enzyme had a 22.6 percent decrease in lipoprotein(a) (protein compounds that carry cholesterol in the blood). LDL also dropped, as did oxidative stress. At the same time, Co-Q10 gave HDL a significant boost. None of these effects were seen in the participants taking the placebo.

Although there are a variety of Co-Q10 formulations on the market, look for soft gel caps. Unlike powdered supplements, gel caps contain Co-Q10 in an oil-based suspension which is considerably more absorbable.

Amino Acids

Amino acids are the "building blocks" of the body. Besides building cells and repairing tissue, they form antibodies to combat invading bacteria and viruses; they are part of the enzyme and hormonal system; they build nucleoproteins (RNA and DNA);

they carry oxygen throughout the body; and they participate in muscle activity. While many amino acids can be manufactured by the body, eight of them (known as essential amino acids) can't be and so they must be provided through food or supplements.

While the three amino acids below are non-essential, if you have heart disease, your body may not be able to make sufficient amounts to keep up with the demands of a compromised cardiovascular system. And if you don't eat much protein or are a vegetarian, it's particularly important to take these amino acids in supplemental form.

Arginine: Arginine is quickly gaining a reputation as the artery-protecting amino acid that boosts nitric oxide levels. As a result, arterial blood vessels relax, permitting improved blood flow to the heart and reducing blood pressure. Some researchers also suggest that the increase in

> ### How Much Should I Take?
>
> Supplements are sold as L-arginine and I recommend taking 1,000 mg. three times a day. But, if you are taking nitroglycerin or any other medication that dilates the blood vessels, avoid taking this

arginine-induced nitric oxide may increase exercise capacity in people with angina.

To test this theory, Polish physicians conducted a double-blind study involving 22 people with stable angina. Each subject took an exercise stress test, which was discontinued when metabolic heart muscle strain was detected. For three days, half the group received a placebo while the others took 1,000 mg. of L-arginine twice daily. When the participants repeated the test, those in the placebo group had increased their exercise time by about one minute. The arginine patients, however, increased their time by nearly three minutes.

According to Johns Hopkins cardiologist Charles J. Lowenstein, nitric oxide also has the power to block the release of inflammatory compounds by cells within the blood vessels. Normally, these cells activate a process that releases packets of molecules into the bloodstream that, like tiny hand grenades, explode and discharge compounds that trigger inflammation. Nitric oxide can move in and target a protein within the endothelial cells called N-ethylmaleimide-Sensitive Factor (NSF) that stops the process from happening by blocking the ability of NSF to push out the molecules.

In addition, some studies have found that arginine lowers cholesterol and opens clogged arteries. In one study, which was published in the journal *Circulation*, patients with high cholesterol who took arginine on a long-term basis experienced a reduction in the thickness of plaque. New evidence also indicates that this amino acid helps to regulate platelet aggregation.

L-Carnitine: L-carnitine may benefit people with cardiomyopathy, angina and congestive heart failure. In one clinical trial, 80 of 160 heart attack patients took 4,000 mg. of L-carnitine a day for one year. Subjects given the L-carnitine showed less mortality and an improved heart rate, rhythm and pressure as well as improved blood lipids.

Controlled research has also shown that people stand a better chance of surviving a heart attack if they are given L-carnitine supplements. And this amino acid has a reputation for increasing exercise capacity. But much of the research on carnitine's impact on exercise in people with congestive heart failure used a modified form of carnitine called propionyl-L-carnitine (PC).

How Much Should I Take?

Most people do not need to supplement their diet with L-carnitine. However, for therapeutic use, the standard dosage is 1,000 to 3,000 mg. per

In one double-blind trail, 500 mg. of PC per day led to a 26 percent increase in exercise capacity after only six months. In other research, patients with congestive heart failure given 1,500 mg. a day had a 21 percent increase in exercise tolerance and a 45 percent increase in oxygen consumption.

Taurine: This amino acid-like nutrient gained attention after a study in the *Japanese Circulation Journal* found it produced a significant improvement in cardiac output and shortness of breath. The study also found that taurine helps regulate the heart beat and maintain cell membrane stability. More recently, Korean researchers discovered that taurine reduced total cholesterol levels by 32 percent, LDL by 37 percent and triglycerides by an impressive 43 percent.

But this amino acid may be particularly important for diabetics at risk for heart disease since they are especially prone to blood clots due to sticky platelets. While the platelets in healthy people normally contain a very high level of taurine, diabetics typically have decreased taurine levels in their blood and in their platelets. But a recent study by Dr. Flavia Franconi of the University of Sassari in Italy discovered that giving diabetics modest supplements of taurine (500 mg. three times a day) reversed the abnormal tendency of their blood platelets to clot.

How Much Should I Take?

If you are a diabetic at high risk for heart disease, I would advise taking 1,500 mg. of taurine a day, in divided doses. However taurine should be taken only under the supervision of a doctor. Unlike most supplements, taurine has a relative narrow divide between therapeutic and toxic doses.

Food sources of taurine include fish and organ meats like liver. However, when taurine levels are depleted by disease or the body's ability to manufacture taurine is inadequate, food sources alone will

How Much Should I Take?

To ensure you're getting all of the heart-healthy advantages fish oil has to offer, take 1,000 mg. of an EPA/DHA fish oil supplement from cold-pressed pure marine lipid every day. Available in capsule form, take them mid-meal to avoid any fishy taste and gassiness that can occur. And always keep your fish oil supplements in the refrigerator since these polyunsaturated oils can go rancid if left at room temperature.

probably not be able to restore adequate taurine levels.

Fish Oil

Even if you don't like fish, you need fish oil. The reason is that fish oil contains eicospentaenoic acid (EPA) and docosahexaenoic acid (DHA), two omega-3 fatty acids that help reduce high blood pressure and modulate many of the mechanisms of atherosclerosis, including inflammation, blood clotting and platelet aggregation (stickiness).

Fish oil may also reduce the chances of dying from a heart attack. One study in the *New England Journal of Medicine* began following 22,000 men with no known heart problems in 1982. In the men who ate fish regularly – one to four times per week – the risk of heart-attack death was as much as 81 percent lower!

Other research shows that fish oil can improve your cholesterol profile. Canadian scientists divided 50 men with high cholesterol into four groups. One group received either a combination of 12,000 mg. of fish oil with 900 mg. of garlic, fish oil alone, garlic alone or a placebo. While the fish oil reduced triglyceride levels by 37.2 percent after 12 weeks, the researchers found that those taking the garlic-fish oil combination had a 34.3 percent reduction in both LDL cholesterol and triglycerides and a 12.2 percent decrease in their total cholesterol. Another study reported that moderate amounts of fish oil – 6,000 mg. a day – lowered triglyceride levels by 30 percent in diabetic adults.

Fish oil is one of the best supplements you can take to support heart health, particularly if you've already suffered a heart attack. But diabetics are often told not to take it in supplemental form because it can raise blood sugar. Recent studies, however, are debunking that theory. In fact, one clinical trial by Harvard researchers even concluded that not only did fish oil have no effect on glucose metabolism, it should be considered an integral part successfully treating diabetes.

Policosanol

Policosanol is the generic name for a mixture of alcohols derived from sugar cane which can lower the production of the cholesterol to more favorable levels. Policosanol also enhances our body's ability to remove and process LDL cholesterol from the blood and cells. In fact, study after study has found that this natural supplement is just as effective as statin drugs.

In one of these studies, a team of German scientists reviewed the literature on placebo-controlled lipid-lowering trials using policosanol and found that, at doses of 10 to 20 mg. per day, policosanol lowers total cholesterol by 17 to 21 percent and LDL cholesterol by 21 to 29 percent. Better yet,

How Much Should I Take?

Most studies have used 5 to 10 mg. of policosanol twice a day. But I recommend starting out with 5 mg. taken once a day at dinnertime. Unlike statin drugs, policosanol can take up to 12 weeks before any results are seen. And early cholesterol testing may show an increase in LDL, but this effect is temporary.

If you have extremely high cholesterol, you can double the dose to 5 mg. twice a day, taken at lunch and dinner.

policosanol raises HDL cholesterol by 8 to 15 percent – more than statin drugs.

In a direct comparison with statin drugs, policosanol also holds its own. In a side-by-side evaluation by Chilean researchers, 10 mg. of policosanol reduced LDL cholesterol by 24 percent compared with 22 percent for Mevacor and 15 percent for Zocor. But, unlike statins, which become increasingly toxic with higher doses, policosanol achieves its maximum effect at very low doses and taking more is neither more effective nor more toxic.

Studies have shown that policosanol is generally safe, but there are a few notes of caution. When policosanol is combined with aspirin, an increased blood-thinning effect occurs. This suggests that policosanol should not be taken with blood-thinning drugs without the supervision of a doctor. Also, some study subjects have experienced mild side effects from policosanol, including insomnia, headache, diarrhea, nervousness and weight loss. These short-term side effects have been reported in less than one percent of the subjects tested. And unlike statin drugs, policosanol has not been shown to have a harmful effect on the liver - the organ that manages the production of cholesterol.

Another concern is that some research indicates that policosanol may have a negative effect on Co-Q10 levels – but these results are preliminary and far from conclusive. However, since supplementing with Co-Q10 is helpful for people with heart disease, some policosanol manufacturers have added CoQ10 to their supplement formulas.

Soy Supplements

For years, soy supplements were recommended to help lower cholesterol. Although the research wasn't conclusive, some researchers believed that the isoflavones in soy could reduce both total cholesterol and LDL. But now, researchers at North Carolina's Wake Forest University have found that, unlike whole soy foods, the isolated soy isoflavones (ISO) in soy supplements don't lower cholesterol levels at all.

The researchers divided 60 menopausal subjects into three groups of 20. The first was fed a milk-based diet likely to lead to atherosclerosis, the second received ISO supplements and the third was fed a diet similar to the first group but with added soy foods. At the end of the study, the group eating the soy food diet had a significantly lower risk of atherosclerosis than those who consumed all of their protein from milk. And those eating the soy had 50 percent lower LDL cholesterol levels than those taking the ISO supplements.

The upshot is that no one really knows for sure if ISO supplements are beneficial or not. Until researchers have clear-cut answers, its far better to get your soy from food instead of simply popping a soy supplement.

REMEMBER . . .

➤ Whenever possible, it's wise to get most of your nutrients through a diet rich in fruits and vegetables.

➤ Taking a multivitamin daily is an important safeguard against disease. But, if you have heart disease, you may need additional nutrients.

➤ Vitamin C is a key nutrient for protecting against atherosclerosis because it inhibits platelet aggregation, prevents the oxidation of LDL cholesterol and lowers CRP.

➤ Vitamin E also lowers CRP and offers exceptional protection against heart attack.

➤ If you have high homocystine levels, make sure you are taking a supplement that provides at least 800 mcg. of folic acid, along with vitamins B-6 and B-12.

➤ Minerals are also important to cardiovascular health, especially calcium, magnesium and selenium. These minerals all work to prevent atherosclerosis.

➤ Low levels of Co-Q10 are implicated in all forms of cardiovascular disease. This important antioxidant should be taken by anyone with heart disease and particularly those taking statin drugs.

➤ Fish oil supplements rich in EPA and DHA can prevent heart attack, lower blood pressure, decrease CRP levels, reduce platelet aggregation and improve your cholesterol profile, making it essential for heart health.

➤ Policosanol is a natural and highly effective alternative to statin drugs.

Chapter 8
HOW HERBS CAN HELP

Medicinal herbs have a time-tested track record for both effectiveness and safety. Made from the leaves, stems, roots, bark, buds and flowers of certain plants, many herbs can still be found in their traditional form – often as teas. But, thanks to modern processing, most herbs are now available as tablets, capsules, powders and tinctures. For the most part, these convenient forms are just as effective as traditional preparations.

Because these plant-based remedies are powerful medicine, always tell your doctor what herbs you are taking, especially if you are scheduled for surgery. A few herbs, like garlic and ginkgo biloba, have been found to interfere with anesthesia or increase the risk of bleeding.

> ## How Much Should I Take?
>
> Both the dried bark and arjuna supplements are available. However, if you're shopping for an arjuna supplement, look for a product that contains one percent arjunolic acid. I've found that 500 mg. three times a day is sufficient to reduce cholesterol levels.

Arjuna: This traditional Ayurvedic herb is a powerful vasodilator that significantly improves the signs and symptoms of cardiomyopathy and angina, as well as heart function.

In the last few years, research on arjuna has exploded. In one study, 58 men with stable angina received either 500 mg. of arjuna every eight hours, a vasodilating drug or a placebo for one week each with a three day washout period in between the treatments. During each treatment, the volunteers took part in treadmill testing. When the researchers compared the data from the three treatment periods, they found that arjuna was just as effective as the drug at increasing exercise tolerance.

Arjuna is also a potent antioxidant and at least one study has shown that it outperforms vitamin E in reducing cholesterol. After dividing 105 patients into three groups, the researchers measured the effects of arjuna, vitamin E or a placebo on cholesterol. No changes were seen in the vitamin E and placebo groups. However, those taking the arjuna had a 12.7 percent decrease in total cholesterol and a 25.6 percent reduction in LDL.

Artichoke Leaf: Taken at high levels, artichoke leaf has also been shown to reduce cholesterol. In one preliminary trial and one controlled trial, use of a standardized artichoke extract was found to lower cholesterol and triglycerides significantly at doses ranging from 900 to 1,920 mg. a day.

> ### How Much Should I Take?
> While all of the studies on artichoke leaf have used fairly high doses of the extract, the typical recommendation is 300 to 640 mg. three times a day for at least six weeks. But if you are allergic to artichokes or have gallstones or other bile-duct obstructions, you should avoid this herb.

While scientists don't really know how artichoke leaves lower cholesterol, some researchers speculate that the herb helps the liver regulate how much cholesterol it makes by boosting bile output. The flavonoids in the plant also prevent LDL oxidation.

Bromelain: Bromelain is a natural blood thinner because it prevents excessive blood platelet stickiness. This may explain the positive reports that bromelain decreases the symptoms of angina. In one preliminary study, 600 cancer patients were receiving 400 to 1,000 mg. of bromelain per day. Among the patients were 14 people who also suffered from angina. In all 14 cases, the angina disappeared within 90 days after starting bromelain.

This pineapple derivative also has an anti-clotting action that may help prevent ischemic stroke and heart attack. Laboratory testing has found that bromelain inhibits platelet-activating factor (PAF), a chemical that signals blood platelets to form clots. Inhibiting PAF short-circuits the entire clotting process and leads to lower blood pressure and reductions in chest pain. Bromelain also breaks down arterial plaques once they have formed.

Bromelain is generally safe and free of side effects when taken in moderate amounts. But one preliminary report indicates that bromelain may increase heart rate. And, because bromelain acts as a blood thinner, talk to your doctor before combining the herb with aspirin or other blood-thinning medications.

Cordyceps: This traditional Chinese medicine (TCM) increases the heart's strength while slowing the heart rate. It also normalizes cardiac arrhythmias. In one clinical trial, over 84 percent of patients

How Much Should I Take?

Although bromelain is usually taken as a digestive aid, if you have atherosclerosis, I advise taking 1,500 to 3,000 mg. a day. However, if you are allergic to pineapple, avoid bromelain supplements.

How Much Should I Take?

The traditional dose is 3,000 to 9,000 mg. taken twice a day in powdered or tincture form.

Although cordyceps has a long history of use, people with hormone-sensitive diseases like breast or prostate cancer should not use it. It should also be avoided if you use anticoagulant drugs, asthma inhalers or have an autoimmune disease.

with cardiac arrhythmia improved following treatment with cordyceps.

According to TCM practitioners, cordyceps also increases the blood supply to the arteries and heart, and lowers blood pressure. And researchers at Mukogawa Women's University in Japan have found that cordyceps contains potent antioxidant properties that may fight free radical oxidation.

A number of studies also show that cordyceps lowers LDL while raising HDL. In addition, one of these studies found that the fungus significantly lowers total cholesterol. What's even better, this time-honored medicine stops the formation of cholesterol plaques by stimulating the activity of macrophages that might otherwise lodge in the artery wall and become a platform for the accumulation of cholesterol.

Fenugreek: The seeds of fenugreek comprise a potent bunch of phytochemicals that may prove beneficial for those with high blood lipids. The most important are compounds known as steroidal saponins that inhibit both cholesterol absorption in the intestines and cholesterol production by the liver. Multiple human trials have found that fenugreek may

How Much Should I Take?

I recommend taking 5,000 to 30,000 mg. of fenugreek with meals three times a day. Although fenugreek is extremely safe, avoid taking more than 100,000 mg. daily since this can cause intestinal upset and nausea.

Talk to your doctor if you are taking an anti-coagulant drug like warfarin or ticlopidine since fenugreek contains coumarin-like substances and the combination may cause bleeding. Some diabetes drugs, especially glipizide, can also adversely interact with fenugreek. However, if you are on insulin, fenugreek may help your medication work more efficiently.

help lower total cholesterol in people with moderate atherosclerosis or those with diabetes.

In one of these trials, 20 adults with high cholesterol levels were assigned to one of two groups. One group consumed 12,500 mg. of fenugreek a day while the other took 18,000 mg. At the end of 30 days, both groups showed improvement. But the group taking the higher dose had significantly lower LDL and total cholesterol levels.

Double-blind trials have also shown that fenugreek lowers triglyceride levels in the blood. In one investigation, diabetic patients took either a powdered fenugreek supplement (50,000 mg.) or a placebo twice a day for 10 days. By the end of the study, all of the patients in the fenugreek group saw a significant reduction in total cholesterol, LDL, lipoprotein(a) and triglycerides. What's more, the fenugreek reduced fasting blood sugar and improved glucose tolerance.

Garlic: Perhaps no other herb has gotten as much press as garlic. This pungent herb lowers blood pressure and improves the elasticity of blood vessel walls. Garlic also reduces cholesterol and acts as a natural blood thinner. Preliminary animal studies suggest that garlic may help lower homocystine levels as well.

How Much Should I Take?

Since there is some evidence that fresh garlic is more potent than garlic supplements, I advise my patients to eat two cloves of garlic a day – something those who like garlic find easy to do. But if you don't like eating garlic or if it bothers your stomach, you can still reap the benefits by taking 2,400 to 7,200 mg. of an aged garlic supplement.

It is important to carefully read the label on all garlic products. Use standardized garlic supplements whenever possible to ensure that you are getting a specified concentration of allicin and other active substances.

In one double-blind cross-over study of 41 moderately hypercholesterolemic men, half took 7,200 mg. of aged garlic every day. The other half were given a placebo. After six months, the groups switched to the other supplement for an additional four months. By the end of the study, the researchers found that the aged garlic supplement reduced total cholesterol by seven percent and LDL cholesterol by 4.6 percent. In addition, there was a 5.5 percent decrease in systolic blood pressure and a modest reduction in diastolic blood pressure. Their conclusion? Aged garlic supplements can benefit people with both moderately high cholesterol and blood pressure.

Garlic supplements have also been found to reduce the size of plaque deposits by nearly 50 percent. In a four-year study of 152 cardiac patients, a daily dose of 900 mg. significantly slowed the development of atherosclerosis. Another study, which measured the flexibility of the aorta of 200 patients, reported that the subjects taking garlic had more flexibility, indicating less atherosclerosis.

The heart-healthy benefits of garlic are due, in large part, to a compound called allicin. This sulfur-rich substance is activated when the clove is crushed and allowed to sit for about 10 minutes. Allicin is then further broken down to a compound called ajoene, which may be the substance that inhibits blockage in blood vessels from clots and atherosclerosis.

Although garlic is generally recognized as safe, it can interact with certain medications. Avoid taking this herb if you are on aspirin therapy or other blood-thinners like warfarin. Garlic may also exaggerate the activity of drugs that inhibit the action of platelets such as indomethacin or dipyridamole. And if you are scheduled for surgery, be sure to let your doctor know that you are taking supplemental garlic. Too much garlic can increase your risk for bleeding during or after surgical procedures.

Ginger: While you may think that ginger belongs in your spice cabinet, this widely-used herb reduces cholesterol levels. In clinical trials conducted in India, 5,000 mg. of dried ginger a day reversed increases in triglycerides and LDL levels, and made blood platelets less sticky and less likely to aggregate – all in as little as

How Much Should I Take?

While most studies use extremely high doses of ginger, I recommend taking 500 mg. of supplemental ginger twice a day.

You can also increase the amount you consume by adding freshly grated ginger to soups, vegetables and stir-fried dishes.

seven days! Another study found that this warming herb lowered total cholesterol and triglycerides by up to 29 percent, lipoprotein(a) by up to 52 percent and LDL levels by up to 58 percent. Impressive, to say the least.

Australian researchers have also discovered that ginger may be more effective than aspirin for preventing blood clots. The researchers looked at whether the chemicals in ginger could inhibit platelet activation in human blood and found that gingerol compounds and their derivatives are even more potent anti-platelet agents than the over-the-counter drug.

Ginger is available in either tablet or capsule form, or as a tea. Side effects are rare, but if taken in excessive doses the herb may cause mild heartburn. Ginger can, however, increase the potency of medications used to prevent blood clots (aspirin, Plavix or Coumadin). If you are taking one of these blood-thinning drugs, you should avoid taking supplemental ginger.

Ginkgo Biloba: Best known as the memory herb, ginkgo biloba is also a powerful weapon against vascular disease. Ginkgo flavone glycosides, which typically make up approximately 24 percent of the extract, are primarily responsible for ginkgo's antioxidant activity and its ability to inhibit platelet aggregation.

This ability, in turn, improves blood flow.

A few years ago, the University of Texas conducted a study on healthy volunteers and patients who had been diagnosed with Type 2 diabetes. By the end of the three month study, the Texas team found that 120 mg. of ginkgo, administered daily, acted as an effective blood thinner.

Ginkgo has also been used by French and German doctors to treat intermittent claudication (leg pain caused by obstructed blood flow related to atherosclerosis). In one 26-week trial, 111 patients with peripheral arterial disease were divided into two groups. All of the patients received a placebo for the first two weeks. Half were then given a standardized ginkgo biloba supplement three times a day (120 mg. total) while the other half continued taking the placebo.

Researchers compared the distance the patients could walk without experiencing pain at the beginning of the study and periodically throughout the trial. After six months, those taking the ginkgo could walk twice as far as those taking the placebo. Other studies have found similar results with increases in pain-free walking up to 500 feet.

Ginkgo is essentially devoid of any serious side effects, but some people (less than one percent) may experience mild gastrointestinal upset. Although no interactions with commonly prescribed drugs are known, ginkgo shouldn't be taken with other blood thinners, either pharmaceutical or herbal.

How Much Should I Take?

I recommend taking 120 to 240 mg. a day. And it's best to take a standardized extract to contain 24 percent ginkgo flavone glycosides and six percent terpene lactones.

But don't expect immediate results. It can take six weeks or more for ginkgo's benefits to appear. After six months, however, the results should be significant.

Green Tea: Although black and oolong tea also confer health benefits, green tea has gained a reputation as a cardiac superstar. Unlike other types of tea, green tea is made from unfermented leaves and contains the highest concentration of polyphenols, leading some researchers to suggest that green tea may be an even more potent antioxidant than vitamin C. In fact, green tea contains roughly 30 to 40 percent polyphenols compared to black tea, which only contains three to 10 percent.

This tasty tea has been shown to mildly lower total cholesterol levels and improve the cholesterol profile in several studies. In one study, 1,371 Japanese men were surveyed on how much green tea they drank per day. Those who drank upwards of ten cups a day had low levels of total cholesterol, LDL and triglycerides, as well as healthy HDL levels, regardless of other dietary considerations. Based on several animal studies, these findings may be due to green tea's ability to block the intestinal absorption of cholesterol and promote its excretion from the body.

How Much Should I Take?

I strongly recommend drinking four to eight cups of green tea a day. But if you'd rather not drink green tea on a regular basis, you can find it in supplement form. Some supplements provide up to 97 percent polyphenol content, which is the equivalent of drinking four cups of tea.

The catechins in green tea may also help protect against heart disease. To test the theory, Dutch researchers analyzed data from the Zutphen Elderly Study, a prospective cohort study of over 800 men, 65-84 years old, beginning in 1985. Health, lifestyle and diet histories were recorded and dietary intakes were analyzed for flavonoid content, specifically for catechins. After 10 years of follow-up, the researchers found that the participants who consumed the most catechins had a 25 percent lower risk of developing atherosclerosis.

Scientists are also looking at green tea's ability to prevent LDL oxidation. And population-based studies indicate that the antioxidant properties of green tea may help prevent atherosclerosis by making platelets less sticky. While the evidence isn't conclusive, it is promising.

Guggul: A resin from the mukul myrrh tree, guggul is a staple in Ayurvedic medicine because of its ability to lower cholesterol

How Much Should I Take?

I advise taking 25 mg. of guggul extract three times a day for a total of 75 mg. daily. Dosage is based on the amount of guggulsterones (the cholesterol-lowering compound in guggul) in the extract and most are standardized to contain 5 to 10 percent of the compound. Like ginkgo, guggul doesn't work quickly. Allow at least 12 weeks before evaluating its effect.

and treat atherosclerosis. One double-blind trial studying the effects of guggul reported that serum cholesterol dropped by 17.5 percent. In another double-blind trial comparing guggul to the drug clofibrate, the average fall in serum cholesterol was slightly greater in the guggul group; moreover, HDL cholesterol rose in 60 percent of people taking guggul, while clofibrate did not elevate HDL at all.

But, doctors at the Medical Hospital and Research Centre in Moradabad, India have found that for guggul to be truly effective, it must be combined with a low-fat diet. In their study, 61 patients with high cholesterol were given 50 mg. of guggulipid or a placebo twice a day. At the same time, all of the subjects were required to eat a diet centered around fruits and vegetables. After 24 weeks, the patients in the guggul group had decreased their total cholesterol by 11.7 percent, LDL by 12.5 percent and triglycerides by 12 percent. The researchers also found that lipid peroxides, a marker of oxidative stress, also declined by 33 percent. As for the subjects in the placebo group, no change was noted in any of the areas measured. But the study didn't end there. After 36 weeks, the researchers found that the lipid-lowering effect of the combination of diet and guggul was just as great as the effect of modern cholesterol-lowering drugs.

The secret to guggul's success are guggulsterones, substances also known as extract isolates ketonic steroid compounds. Guggulsterones not only prevent LDL oxidation, they also reduce the stickiness of platelets. What's more, scientists from the Southern California University of Health Sciences reported on a clinical trial showing that guggul also offers anti-inflammatory properties.

Hawthorn: If you could rely on just one herb for heart disease, this would be it. Rich in antioxidants, French researchers recently found that an extract made from the tops and flowers of the herb could significantly reduce LDL oxidation.

Clinical trials have also confirmed that hawthorn leaf and flower extracts are beneficial for people with early-stage congestive heart failure. In one study, patients with congestive heart failure taking 160–900 mg. of hawthorn extract per day for eight weeks showed improved quality of life, including greater ability to exercise without shortness of breath and exhaustion.

But one of the most remarkable studies of hawthorn involved 3,600 patients. The subjects were treated three times a day with

How Much Should I Take?

It's best to take Hawthorn as a liquid extract and I recommend taking one to three teaspoons two to three times a day.

Hawthorn is slow acting and may take one to two months for maximum effects to be seen. However, it appears to be safe and should be considered a long-term therapy.

300 mg. of hawthorn standardized to 2.2 percent flavonoids. Although it was an observational study and not a placebo-controlled trial, the eight-week results were impressive: Heart palpitations dropped from an average of 40 percent to 18 percent, edema was reduced from 50 percent to 13 percent and the overall symptom score was lowered from nine to three. The authors noted that hawthorn provided a significant overall benefit for patients with the symptoms of congestive heart failure.

Hawthorn contains large amounts of flavonoids that stabilize capillaries and strengthen weak blood vessels. Hawthorn is also a wonderful heart tonic since it helps treat elevated cholesterol levels and slightly lowers blood pressure. And one study has found that hawthorn leaf and flower extract may help those with stable angina. If that weren't enough, this herb acts as a natural calcium channel blocker and an ACE (angiotensin converting enzyme) inhibitor.

Pycnogenol: Pycnogenol, a standardized extract of French maritime pine bark, is one of the family of flavonoids known as oligomeric proanthocyanidins or OPCs. And, until recently, its biggest claim to fame was as an antioxidant. But researchers at the University of Arizona recently found that Pycnogenol reduces platelet activity, lowers high blood pressure, relaxes artery constriction and improves circulation. Other studies have found that Pycnogenol dilates small blood vessels in people with heart disease using doses as low as 100 mg. a day.

How Much Should I Take?

Most recent studies have used doses that range from 150 to 360 mg. But I've seen evidence that doses as low as 50 to 100 mg. can offer heart-healthy benefits.

Although generally considered safe, Pycnogenol can upset the stomach, so make sure you take it with meals.

But Pycnogenol's benefits don't stop there. During a study comparing Pycnogenol to horse chestnut seed extract's ability to treat chronic venous insufficiency, German researchers accidentally discovered that Pycnogenol also reduces cholesterol. Of the 40 people taking part in their study, those taking the OPC had a 13 percent drop in LDL and total cholesterol was reduced by 19.7 percent. Other studies suggest that Pycnogenol also raises HDL slightly.

Because of its high antioxidant content, Pycnogenol acts as a free radical scavenger. It's so effective that some scientists suggest it may outpace vitamin E's antioxidant capabilities.

Quercetin: Population studies have found that people with high intakes of quercetin tend to have lower rates of heart disease. One reason is that this antioxidant has the ability to dilate blood vessels and reduce plaque formation.

How Much Should I Take?

Although I recommend that my patients take 200 to 500 mg. of quercetin two to three times per day, talk to your doctor before taking this supplement.

Women who are pregnant or those taking estradiol should not use quercetin. Neither should people taking the immune suppressant drug cyclosporine or calcium channel blockers.

When a blood vessel is injured (by disease or high blood pressure), specialized clean-up cells called macrophages accumulate at the site of the injury. Macrophages contain large amounts of cholesterol which can accumulate and harden into plaques. Quercetin slows the series of chemical reactions that cause large macrophages to cluster on artery walls, reducing the risk of plaque formation. In one study, quercetin reduced the size of atherosclerotic lesions by 46 percent and LDL oxidation by 48 percent.

This herb has a special relationship with vitamin C: Quercetin regenerates oxidized vitamin C and vitamin C can bring quercetin back to life. As a result, both supplements are often taken together.

Red Clover: While menopause increases a woman's risk for developing cardiovascular disease, the isoflavones in red clover have been associated with a sizeable increase in HDL cholesterol, leading some researchers to suggest that red clover may help protect pre- and postmenopausal women against heart disease.

> ## How Much Should I Take?
>
> The most recommended dose is 500 mg. two to six times a day for menopausal symptoms. But, since the research into red clover's role in reducing heart disease is still in the early stages, no amount has been established for the treatment of heart disease.

Interestingly, a recent study also found that menopausal women who took 50 mg. of supplemental red clover a day experienced a significant improvement in arterial compliance (a measure of the strength and resilience of the arterial walls) and, as a result, lower blood pressure. Arterial compliance diminishes during menopause and may increase a woman's risk for heart disease.

Although non-fermented red clover supplements are relatively safe, this herb can interact with certain medications used to control heart disease. Check with your doctor if you are taking an anticoagulant like heparin, platelet-inhibiting drugs or blood thinning medications like warfarin.

REMEMBER . . .

➤ Herbs, while generally safe, are potent medicines.

➤ Many herbal remedies are just as effective as prescription drugs. For example, arjuna works as well as vasodilating drugs for increasing exercise tolerance. And guggul is just as effective as some cholesterol- lowering medications.

➤ Along with their primary action, many of the herbs taken for heart disease are potent antioxidants. As such, they also fight free radical damage that contributes to artery damage and LDL oxidation.

➤ Unlike prescription or over-the-counter drugs, herbs often take weeks or months before their benefits can be measured.

➤ Along with using supplements, some heart-healthy herbs like garlic, ginger and green tea can also be included in your diet.

➤ If you suffer from congestive heart failure or angina, make sure to include hawthorn in your treatment plan.

➤ Whenever possible, choose a standardized herbal preparation.

➤ Make sure to tell your doctor what herbs you are taking. Some herbal remedies can interact with other medications or can cause adverse reactions during surgery.

➤ Be careful when combining herbal therapies that have similar actions. Some can cause negative effects if taken together.

Chapter 9
NATURAL ALTERNATIVES TO SURGERY

What if your heart disease has progressed to the point where diet, exercise and supplements just aren't enough? Some patients with severe heart disease may suffer from unrelenting angina. Or perhaps they can't walk half a block without experiencing exhaustion and breathlessness. These patients need immediate therapy. But is surgery the only answer?

Fortunately, there are two very powerful alternatives. Unlike bypass surgery or angioplasty, these therapies aren't invasive and involve no hospitalization, sedation or trauma to the body. And, unlike drugs, they are safe and don't carry the risk of side effects. Best of all, they work.

EDTA Chelation Therapy

EDTA chelation is a therapy by which repeated administrations of a weak synthetic amino acid (EDTA, ethylenediamine tetra-acetic acid) gradually reduce atherosclerotic plaque and other mineral deposits throughout the cardiovascular system by literally dissolving them away. This alternative to angioplasty and bypass surgery has frequently been compared to a natural "Roto-Rooter" because it removes plaque and returns the arterial system to a smooth, healthy, pre-atherosclerotic state.

When EDTA is slowly infused into the blood-stream, it binds with minerals like calcium, iron or lead and carries them to the kidneys where they are excreted. Although some minerals (like calcium) are required for optimum health, when they build up in the body, they can speed up the oxidation process. By removing excess minerals through chelation, free radicals are kept under control and atherosclerosis is slowed.

EDTA chelation attacks atherosclerosis in other ways too. It dissolves excess calcium from the arterial walls, making them more responsive and better able to dilate. This action alone can improve blood flow and general circulation. It also has blood-thinning effects and discourages the formation of blood clots. And it's a powerful antioxidant that limits free radical damage.

EDTA was synthesized in Germany in 1935, and first used in industry as a chelating agent, as an anticoagulant for clinical laboratory use and as a treatment for lead poisoning. But in 1955, Dr. Norman Clarke, then Director of Research of Providence Hospital in Detroit, Michigan, reported on his use of intravenous EDTA to dissolve what he referred to as "metastatic calcium" (calcium deposits in the arteries, joints and kidneys) with generally favorable results.

Among 283 patients treated by Dr. Clarke and his colleagues from 1956 to 1960, 87 percent showed improvement. Heart patients got better and patients with blocked arteries in their legs, particularly those with diabetes, avoided amputation. Since then, hundreds of papers have been published on the effects of chelation therapy in a variety of chronic diseases, with the vast majority reporting favorable results.

But in spite of its obvious benefit to heart patients, EDTA fell out of favor in the mid-1960s for two reasons. First, profitable surgery for heart and vessel disease was on the rise. Second, the patent on EDTA (held by Abbott Laboratories) expired, so there was no financial interest for drug companies to fund any research. Fortunately, a small group of practicing physicians

Did you know?

EDTA chelation is so effective at removing unwanted minerals and metals from the blood, it has been the standard FDA-approved treatment for lead, mercury, aluminum and cadmium poisoning for more than 50 years.

who used EDTA chelation founded an organization in 1973 called the American College for the Advancement of Medicine to educate both consumers and doctors about the benefits of EDTA chelation therapy.

Proven Benefits

The first randomized, double-blind, controlled clinical trial of EDTA chelation therapy for the treatment of atherosclerosis was conducted by the University Hospital in Heidelberg, West Germany. That study compared EDTA chelation therapy to the platelet inhibitor bencyclan, a drug widely prescribed in Europe to treat atherosclerosis.

A total of 48 patients were treated – 24 in the bencyclan group and 24 in the EDTA group. Only patients with peripheral vascular disease who could not walk 200 meters without the pain of claudication (caused by impaired blood supply) were included in the study. Pain-free walking distance was measured before, during and after therapy on a treadmill. Those in the EDTA group were given treatments five days a week for four weeks, for a total of 20 treatments while the rest of the subjects took only bencyclan. By the end of the study, the EDTA group showed a 250 percent increase in pain-free

Safe, Effective and Painless!

EDTA chelation is administered in a doctor's office, usually once or twice a week. You sit in a recliner and an IV is inserted into a vein in your arm (the only part of the treatment that may be uncomfortable). Then you simply sit back and relax while the EDTA slowly circulates through the miles of blood vessels in your body.

Each treatment takes about three hours, and a complete course is between 20 and 30 treatments. Patients with chronic heart problems may, after the initial series of treatments, continue their therapy on a once a month basis.

walking distance compared to only a 60 percent increase in the bencyclan group.

It's not unusual for physicians who regularly prescribe EDTA chelation to encounter heart disease patients who have failed all the standard treatments but who make remarkable - even unbelievable - recoveries once EDTA has been given. In fact, many patients on waiting lists for bypass surgery have found they didn't need surgery following a series of EDTA chelation treatments.

One particular study found that when 65 patients who had been on the waiting list for bypass surgery for an average of 6 months were treated with EDTA chelation therapy, the symptoms in 89 percent of them improved so much that they canceled their surgery. In the same study, 27 patients who had been recommended for limb amputation due to poor peripheral circulation, underwent EDTA chelation therapy, which saved 24 of the limbs.

Not all of the studies on EDTA have reached positive conclusions however. Several studies have found no apparent benefit and two, in particular, are often cited by critics. But a closer analysis of these studies revealed problems with both the controls and the interpretation of the data.

In the first study, Danish researchers gave 153 patients with claudication either 20 intravenous EDTA treatments or 20 placebo treatments. While all of the patients were measured for pain-free walking distance before and after treatment, the researchers only selected 30 of the participants for additional testing, which included an angiogram. Given the limited number of clinical tests and the subjective nature of the study, it's impossible to measure any definitive improvement.

The second study, which came from New Zealand, also concluded that EDTA offered no benefit to heart patients. But the raw data told a different story. Upon closer inspection, it was found that 26 percent of the EDTA-treated patients achieved an improvement of greater than 100 percent in walking distance compared with only 12 percent of the "placebo" controls. Among nonsmokers or smokers who had quit, 66 percent of the EDTA-treated group increased their walking distance an average of 86 percent compared with 45 percent of the controls, who improved by just 56 percent. Reduced blood flow, as measured by the ankle/brachial index, was found in six percent of the EDTA-treated patients and 35 percent of the controls. Although the authors of these studies reached negative conclusions, in fact, their data actually supported the use of EDTA chelation!

Oral EDTA Chelation

Another option is oral EDTA, which has been used for at least as long as its intravenous cousin. Clinical experience suggests that oral chelation provides many, but not all, of the benefits of IV therapy. Overall, the differences in benefits are more those of degree, speed, convenience and cost per dose than of quality.

Intravenous EDTA chelation has a direct and powerful effect on the body almost instantaneously. Not as convenient as swallowing a few capsules of oral EDTA per day, an IV EDTA session usually lasts several hours, during which about 1,500 to 3,000 mg. of EDTA (plus vitamin C and other nutrients) are administered. Typical candidates for IV chelation are people who have been diagnosed with serious atherosclerosis, symptoms of vascular occlusion or significant calcification of tissues. A series of needed sessions of IV EDTA will cost about $2,000 to $4,000. But for patients with less severe forms of heart disease, oral EDTA may be appropriate and is significantly less costly – about $15 to $40 per month, depending on one's intake.

About 15 percent of an oral dose of EDTA is absorbed into the bloodstream, compared with 100 percent of an IV dose. Yet, due to continuous daily intake, the amounts add up and can definitely achieve similar benefits compared with IV chelation.

Oral EDTA is appropriate for people whose condition does not demand prompt attention. It's especially desirable for preventing or delaying the onset of the many complications of atherosclerotic plaque buildup, including heart disease, heart attack, stroke, high blood pressure, peripheral vascular disease, mental decline and impotence.

So why would anyone opt for an invasive procedure like angioplasty or bypass when a safe and effective alternative exists for restoring normal or near-normal arterial function? In my opinion,

POTENTIAL BENEFITS OF EDTA CHELATION

Prevents cholesterol deposits
Reduces blood cholesterol levels
Lowers high blood pressure
Avoids bypass surgery
Avoids angioplasty
Reserves digitalis toxicity
Removes calcium from atherosclerotic plaques
Dissolves intra-arterial blood clots
Normalizes cardiac arrhythmias
Has an anti-aging effect
Reduces excessive heart contractions
Increases intracellular potassium
Reduces heart irritability
Improves heart function
Removes mineral and deposits
Dissolves kidney stones
Reduces serum iron levels
Reduces heart valve calcification
Reduces varicose veins
Heals calcified necrotic ulcers
Reduces intermittent claudication

Improves vision in diabetic retinopathy
Decreases macular degeneration
Dissolves small cataracts
Eliminates heavy metal toxicity
Makes arterial walls more flexible
Prevents osteoarthritis
Reduces rheumatoid arthritis symptoms
Lowers diabetics' insulin needs
Reduces Alzheimer-like symptoms
Reverses senility
Reduces stroke/heart attack after-effects
Prevents cancer
Improves memory
Reverses diabetic gangrene
Restores impaired vision
Detoxifies snake and spider venoms

Adapted from Walker M., Gordon G., Douglass W.C. *The Chelation Answer*

EDTA should be the first line of treatment, with invasive surgical procedures as the last-resort alternative, not the other way around.

Enhanced External Counterpulsation (EECP)

Enhanced external counterpulsation, or EECP for short, is an idea that dates back to the 1950's. Developed by a Harvard University researcher named Harry Soroff as a treatment for angina, EECP is a mechanical system that actually squeezes the blood out of the lower extremities and up toward the heart. The result is increased circulation and reduced chest pain.

But, although Asian countries quickly embraced this new, non-invasive technology, EECP didn't get much attention in America until recently – after dozens of studies supported its use. In fact, research shows that 80 percent of patients experienced significant improvement following EECP treatment, many experiencing a complete end of symptoms.

In the largest such study to date, seven major research institutions (including Harvard, Yale and Columbia Universities) cooperated in a groundbreaking clinical study that was later reported in the *Journal of the American College of Cardiology*. Researchers found that patients used less medication, had fewer angina attacks, and were able to exercise longer without pain or fatigue after receiving EECP treatment. The study confirmed a number of previous studies that had found EECP to objectively improve the coronary status of patients suffering from angina.

In an attempt to evaluate the longer term benefits of the therapy, an investigation was conducted by the University of Pittsburgh School of Public Health that looked at EECP patients six months and one year following treatment. Researchers found that patients not only maintained the gains they made during treatment, but continued to improve after treatment ended. In other words, patients continued to get better long after treatment ended.

How does EECP compare to surgery? An important breakthrough study by researchers at the State University of New York at Stony Brook compared the long-term benefits of EECP to angioplasty and bypass surgery. Researchers found that five-year outcomes for EECP patients were virtually the same as for patients who had angioplasty, bypass surgery, or both. The study confirmed that EECP is an effective long-term therapy for patients with coronary artery disease.

In a recent issue of *Cardiology*, investigators report that EECP works even better in patients who have not yet had invasive treatment for angina. Among patients participating in the International EECP Patient Registry who received EECP as first-line therapy (instead of receiving it only after other treatments failed), 89 percent experienced an immediate improvement in angina and 84 percent reported that the improvement lasted at least six months. This compares to a 79 percent improvement rate with EECP among patients who had already received invasive treatments.

EECP vs. Surgery

EECP has numerous advantages over traditional cardiac surgery:

- Non-invasive
- Outpatient
- Low risk
- No medication
- No recuperation time
- No side effects
- Patients report increased energy after treatment

How It Works

While the exact mechanism of this therapy is the subject of much speculation, EECP appears to have two potentially beneficial actions on the heart. First, the milking action of the leg cuffs increases the blood flow to the coronary arteries. (The coronary arteries, unlike other arteries in the body, receive their blood flow after each heartbeat instead of during each heartbeat. EECP, effectively, "pumps" blood into the coronary arteries.) Second, by its deflating action just as the heart begins to beat, EECP creates something like a sudden vacuum in the arteries, which reduces the work of the heart muscle in pumping blood into the arteries. Both of these actions have long been known to reduce cardiac ischemia (the lack of oxygen to the heart muscle) in patients with coronary artery disease.

Put The Squeeze On Heart Disease

EECP is a painless, non-invasive treatment that uses a series of inflatable cuffs – much like blood pressure cuffs. These cuffs inflate and deflate in time with your heartbeat, stimulating increased circulation back to your heart. This enhanced circulatory flow helps to develop a network of new vessels that detour around blocked or narrowed arteries, and deliver more oxygen-rich blood to the heart.

The Long-Lasting Benefits

Several studies conducted at leading university medical centers have shown that patients who undergo a course of EECP experience significant benefits:

- They have fewer episodes of angina
- The episodes of angina are less intense
- They need less anti-angina medication
- They can walk farther without experiencing angina
- They can resume work and enjoy more social activities

It's an appropriate alternative to angioplasty, bypass or grafting and laser revascularization for patients with angina. In fact, some doctors consider EECP "nature's bypass." And, this therapy is safe for people with pacemakers, diabetes, kidney or lung disease, or other conditions that may increase the risk of invasive procedures. In fact, EECP is considered so safe that it's the only non-pharmacologic, non-invasive treatment approved by the FDA for angina and congestive heart failure.

The treatment consists of 35 one-hour treatments over the course of seven weeks with the patient on a Monday through Friday regimen. During EECP therapy, the patient lies on a bed and pressure cuffs are attached to the calves, lower thighs and upper thighs. The cuffs inflate and deflate, gradually building to full pressure while the machine works with the heart's rhythms. The patient's heart rate and rhythm are constantly measured during the process.

Most patients tolerate the therapy with little discomfort. The common complaints include mild headache, mild dizziness, fatigue or muscle aches, but these effects are temporary and the vast majority of patients never experience any ill effects. Better yet, unlike surgery or other medical procedures, patients undergoing EECP therapy don't experience any long-term side effects.

Why Your Doctor May Not Tell You About EECP

Despite that fact that EECP therapy is FDA-approved, you probably won't hear much about it from your cardiologist. Why? First of all, EECP doesn't pay well. A series of 35 treatments costs $5,000 to $6,000 dollars. That's not chicken feed, but keep in mind that we're talking about 35 hours of therapy over 7 weeks, which involves not only the doctor's time but also the time of office staff and nursing personnel. Compared to an invasive procedure like angioplasty, it simply isn't profitable.

Then there's the fact that, to accommodate patients for EECP, cardiologists would not only have to purchase expensive equipment, but would have to radically change the organization of their offices, their office staff and their space.

Finally, and most importantly, EECP has nothing in common with what cardiologists do. Cardiologists study and treat the heart – they stress it, image it, measure it, pace it, shock it, stent it, ablate it, revascularize it and bathe it in drugs. What they do takes years of specialized training and expertise, millions of dollars of high-tech equipment, and tremendous manual dexterity – and it brings them significant prestige, even within the medical community.   Now they're supposed to drop all that? Hardly. So it will likely be up to you to broach the subject.

If your doctor discourages you from pursuing EECP, make sure he or she gives you a good reason (you don't have the sort of angina that would benefit from EECP or your coronary artery disease is of the type that requires revascularization). Good reasons would not include: it's unproven, it doesn't work, its voodoo or "I've never heard of it."

REMEMBER . . .

➤ There are safe, natural, non-invasive alternatives to surgery.

➤ EDTA chelation therapy can reduce atherosclerotic plaque, making it an effectivce alternative to angioplasty and bypass surgery.

➤ EDTA also dissolves excess calcium and has blood thinning effects.

➤ Intravenous EDTA is a painless treatment conducted in the doctor's office.

➤ Oral EDTA is another option. Although this form of therapy doesn't work as quickly as intravenous EDTA, it offers many of the same benefits and is much less costly. It is especially useful for less serious forms of heart disease.

➤ EECP is an excellent alternative to bypass surgery for treating angina. It also boosts circulation and exercise capacity.

➤ EECP works by increasing blood flow to the heart and acts like a vacuum in the arteries to reduce the heart's workload.

➤ Many doctors either aren't familiar with these alternatives or discount them. Unless your doctor can give you a solid medical reason why you aren't a good candidate for either EDTA chelation or EECP, seek a second opinion from an integrative physician.

Chapter 10

HOW COMPLIMENTARY MEDICINE KEEPS YOU YOUNG AT HEART

There are many treatments used to treat cardiovascular disease that fall outside the realm of conventional medicine – many of which we've already discussed. But there's one more class of treatments that can support a healthy diet, exercise and heart-healthy supplements. They can also augment conventional treatment, if that's the path you decide to take.

Complementary and alternative medicine, also known as CAM, has gained enormous popularity and acceptance among patients over the last fifteen years. In 1990, Americans made an estimated 425 million visits to an alternative health practitioner – more than they made to primary care physicians. Today, one in three people have used a CAM therapy.

In a world of five minute doctor visits, insurance-dictated treatment plans, HMOs and spiraling health costs, a growing number of informed healthcare consumers are open to trying alternative medical treatments. More importantly, they are demanding to be treated as a person – not simply as a diagnosis – by their health care practitioners.

Mainstream medicine is finally beginning to catch on to the fact that CAM is good medicine. The realization that conventional medicine (antibiotics, prescription drugs and invasive surgery) can't solve all of America's health problems has led nearly one-third of American medical schools – among them Harvard, Yale, John's Hopkins and Georgetown Universities – to adopt courses in alternative medicine. In fact, CAM has become so well accepted that 18 percent of Fortune 500 companies offer alternative medicine as part of their healthcare compensation packages.

One reason CAM therapies are becoming more popular is the fact that they treat the whole person – mind, body and spirit – and not just the physical ailment. This approach is often referred to as "holistic." In other words, these therapies look at illness and its prevention and treatment, in terms of the unique individual rather than just a collection of symptoms. CAM therapies also acknowledge the body's ability to heal itself. The treatments themselves may not "cure" your disease – but they will help restore the body's own self-healing ability. As Voltaire said, "The art of medicine consists of amusing the patient while Nature cures the disease."

Finding a CAM Practitioner

- Many states have regulatory agencies or licensing boards for certain types of practitioners. They may be able to provide you with information regarding practitioners in your area.

- Contact a professional organization for the type of practitioner you are seeking. Often, professional organizations have standards of practice and may provide referrals.

- Ask if it is possible to have a brief consultation in person or by phone with the practitioner. This will give you a chance to speak with the practitioner directly. The consultation may or may not involve a charge.

- After you select a practitioner, make a list of questions to ask at your first visit. What benefits can you expect? Are there any risks? How long will I need to undergo therapy?

- Come to the first visit prepared to answer questions about your health history, as well as prescription medicines, vitamins and other supplements you may take.

CAM therapies include not only the remedies I've already covered in this book, they also encompass more "exotic" treatments, including acupuncture, acupressure, aromatherapeutic massage, osteopathy and reflexology. While these therapies can have a positive impact on many aspects of heart disease, one of the greatest benefits you'll experience is the power to take charge of your own health.

Acupuncture

Just about everyone has heard of acupuncture these days, but few know how this ancient medical therapy really works. Or that it can be an effective treatment for angina and high blood pressure.

> ## HEART SMART TIP
> Cardiovascular disorders that respond well to acupuncture include:
> - Angina
> - Cardiac ischemia
> - Heart rate variability
> - High blood pressure

The traditional form of acupuncture is part of the wider system of Traditional Chinese Medicine (TCM) and has been practiced in China for thousands of years. The fundamental principal of acupuncture is that there are two interactive qualities in nature called "yin" and "yang," which interweave with each other both in the universe and within each person. Good health depends on maintaining the balance between the two. If the balance is disturbed, the result is disease.

Practitioners believe that by influencing "chi," the life force or energy that flows through the body in the blood vessels and in a set of energetic pathways known as meridians which are linked to various organs, they can balance yin and yang. The result is health.

Situated along these meridians are 500 recognized acupuncture points, of which about 100 are commonly used. Generally, these are sites where the meridian runs close to the surface of the body. Hair-thin acupuncture needles can be inserted into these points to rebalance the flow of chi when it is disturbed. Once the needles are in place, they can be stimulated either by hand or electrically to maximize the effect.

Not surprisingly, most Western doctors have trouble with the concept of manipulating chi. But they can't ignore acupuncture's heart healthy benefits. Acupuncture treatments have reduced angina and lowered blood pressure in some patients and, in certain instances, have effectively treated cardiac ischemia which is caused by an inadequate supply of blood to the heart muscle cells. Other research has found that acupuncture can regulate heart rate.

One animal experiment, conducted at China's Norman Bethune University of Medical Sciences, found that manipulating certain acupuncture points not only lowered blood pressure in mice, it also had a positive impact on the levels of five trace elements, including two which are critical for heart health – calcium and magnesium. Several other studies have found that, in addition to lowering blood pressure, acupuncture also has a blood-thinning effect.

Human studies show a similar effect. In one recent clinical trial, 87 hypertensive patients experienced a significant decrease in their systolic blood pressure after being treated with acupuncture. A smaller study found that acupuncture can also reduce diastolic pressure in patients with high blood pressure.

Modern doctors have speculated that acupuncture's heart healthy effects probably come via the endocrine system, since this

> ## Safety Alert!
> The risks of acupuncture are small when treatment is conducted by a qualified practitioner – much lower than those of prescription drugs.
>
> Always choose a qualified acupuncturist. Some states, such as California, New York and Florida, require that acupuncturists become licensed. However, if you don't live in a state that requires licensing, check with either the American Academy of Medical Acupuncture or the National Commission for the Certification of Acupuncturists for a list of certified practitioners.

system not only releases endorphins (the body's natural painkillers), but is responsible for regulating blood pressure, heart rate and inflammation. To test this theory, a team of researchers at the University of California-Irvine and Shanghai Medical University in China increased the levels of a chemical called bradykinin in a group of cats. Bradykinin is produced when the body reacts to infections and, in general, works against the relaxing effects of the endorphin system. The chemical triggers inflammation, raises blood pressure, and makes the heart pump harder and faster.

Tiny electric probes that simulate acupuncture needles in the lab reduced bradykinin levels when the researchers applied the probes to the nerve endings (determined by Chinese acupuncture maps) related to heart disease. The reduced bradykinin levels quickly resulted in lower blood pressure and allowed the heart to pump less strenuously.

But these effects disappeared when the researchers injected naloxone (which inhibits the brain's endorphin system) into the bloodstream. Since naloxone blocks nerve cells in the endorphin system, the scientists concluded that acupuncture was doing its work by stimulating the body's natural endorphins.

What To Expect

Acupuncture therapy usually involves a series of weekly or biweekly treatments in an outpatient setting. A series of treatments (up to 20) is fairly common.

Acupuncture practitioners, like medical doctors, each have their own individual style and way of structuring an office visit. But, in general, an acupuncture visit lasts about an hour. Like a visit to your doctor, an acupuncture visit includes an exam and an assessment of your current condition, the treatment itself and a discussion afterward to suggest self-care tips. During the acupuncture treatment, the practitioner uses disposable sterilized, individually wrapped stainless steel needles. The amount of pain felt when the needles are inserted varies from person to person, but most people only experience mild discomfort.

Before you embark on a course of therapy, however, ask how many treatments will be required. It may not be possible for the acupuncturist to give you a precise number, but he or she should be able to give you a rough estimate. In general, while you may see some improvement after about five visits, it can often take ten or more sessions before you notice a difference. If there hasn't been any effect after a dozen visits, you may be one of the very few people for whom acupuncture isn't an effective treatment.

Acupressure

Although not as well-known as acupuncture, acupressure is rapidly gaining acceptance as a safe, non-invasive form of care. Sometimes referred to as shiatsu massage, acupressure very similar to acupuncture. But instead of inserting needles, acupressure involves using the fingers, thumbs, palms and heels of the hand to apply pressure and stimulate specific points along the meridians of the body.

To see what effect acupressure may have on the cardiovascular system, a pair of researchers from the Faculty of Health Sciences in Linkoping, Sweden conducted a study of 24 healthy male volunteers between the ages of 20 and 36. Their results, which appeared in a recent issue of *Complementary Therapies in Medicine*, showed marked changes in arterial pressure, heart rate and the amount of blood flow to the skin in those receiving acupressure, leading the researchers to conclude that these non-invasive stimulation techniques may be a "low-risk and cost-effective" form of care.

During their study, the subjects were divided into three groups of eight. One group received active stimulation consisting of pressure on acupoints; the second received active stimulation via stroking along the meridians; and the third received controlled stimulation. Stimulation was performed by way of a 15-centimeter long dental instrument with a two-millimeter ball-point at each end.

In the pressure group, 24 classical acupoints were stimulated in order using firm pressure and a gliding movement across the acupoints. In the stroking group, the acupoints of 13 meridians were stimulated by stroking with the tool along the meridians in the direction of the flow (according to traditional Chinese medicine). The stimulation in the control group was achieved with very light pressure along 24 non-acupoints within an inch of the acupoints in the pressure group.

A variety of measurements were taken while the subjects were stimulated, including heart rate, systolic arterial pressure, diastolic arterial pressure, mean arterial pressure and skin blood flow. Data on skin blood flow, arterial pressure and heart rate were recorded once every minute, from 20 minutes before stimulation to 30 minutes after. All measurements were taken by a researcher who was blinded to the type of treatment the subjects received.

Results of the treatment showed dramatic cardiovascular changes in the acupressure group. Heart rate, for instance, decreased an average of seven beats per minute in the group receiving acupressure, compared to five beats for the stroking group and just one beat per minute in the control group. Similar changes in arterial pressure and skin blood flow were seen in the pressure group, but not in the stroking or control groups.

Based on their observations, the researchers concluded that applying pressure to acupoints "can significantly influence the cardiovascular system." Non-invasive stimulation techniques like acupressure, they believe, "could be a low-risk and cost-effective treatment," particularly in areas where acupuncture needles are difficult to obtain.

Aromatherapeutic Massage

Aromatherapeutic massage can be defined as the art and science of combining therapeutic touch with naturally extracted aromatic essences from plants to balance, harmonize and promote the health of body, mind and spirit. As a holistic medicine, aromatherapeutic massage is both a preventative approach as well as an active treatment during acute and chronic stages of disease. It's a natural, non-invasive treatment system designed to affect the

Safety Alert!

Aromatherapy, by itself, can be self-administered. But essential oils are highly concentrated and can be harmful if not used carefully. By treating essential oils as medicines, you will be well on your way to safely enjoying the many benefits that aromatherapy can offer.

- Essential oils should never be used undiluted on the skin. Always dilute them in a carrier oil like almond or grapeseed oil.

- Some oils can cause sensitization or allergic reactions in some individuals. When using a new oil for the first time, place a small amount of the diluted essential oil on the inside of your forearm and apply a bandage. Wait 24 hours to see if there is any reaction.

- Not all essential oils are suitable for use in aromatherapy. Wormwood, pennyroyal, onion, camphor, horseradish, wintergreen, rue, bitter almond and sassafras are some of the essential oils that should only be used by a qualified aromatherapy practitioner, if ever.

- Essential oils should not be taken internally.

whole person – not just the symptom or disease – and to assist the body's natural ability to balance, regulate, heal and maintain itself by the correct use of essential oils.

Essential oils that are inhaled into the lungs are believed to offer both psychological and physical benefits; not only does the aroma of the natural essential oil stimulate the brain to trigger a reaction, but the natural constituents (naturally occurring chemicals) of the essential oil are drawn into the lungs and can also supply physical benefit. Oils that are applied to the skin are believed to be absorbed into the bloodstream. The components of the various oils are believed to aid in a variety of health conditions, including cardiovascular health.

While a plain massage can reduce stress that can contribute to heart disease, an aromatherapeutic massage can lower blood pressure and improve blood circulation without putting additional strain on the heart. It helps the flow of blood through the veins and also stimulates the nerves which control the blood vessels.

HEART SMART TIP

Turn Your Nose Up To Hypertension

Work carried out by Dr. Gary Schwartz, Professor of Psychology and Psychiatry at Yale University, also found that the aromas of some essential oils *by themselves* reduced blood pressure. The scent of spiced apple, for example, was found to reduce blood pressure by an average of three to five points in healthy volunteers.

Other essential oils that may help lower blood pressure include:

- Chamomile
- Marjoram
- Clary Sage
- Rose
- Cypress
- Rosewood
- Lavender
- Ylang-Ylang

Aromatherapeutic massage has the added benefit of relaxing tense muscles and tight connective tissues which may have been constricting blood vessels, thus enabling blood to flow more freely.

In one small pilot study conducted by the Natural Health Centre in Lancashire, UK, 20 patients were divided into two groups. The first group received five 45 minute aromatherapy treatments using grapeseed carrier oil containing one drop of each of ylang-ylang, clary sage and marjoram essential oil over a six week period. The second group received the same massage but without the essential oils. At the end of the treatment period, the results revealed that seven people in the treatment group and six in the control group experienced a reduction in their blood pressure. But those in the aromatherapy group also saw an improvement in their pulse rate – an effect that wasn't experienced by the patients in the control group. The study's authors concluded that overall blood pressure readings in both groups improved significantly, indicating that this type of tactile treatment can have a beneficial effect on the raised arterial blood pressure.

HEART SMART TIP

Massage Away Atherosclerosis

A regular massage with juniper and lemon may help to break down fatty deposits. Massage with the essential oils of peppermint, lavender, rose and marjoram may help strengthen the heart.

What To Expect

The first appointment generally begins with the massage therapist asking what prompted you to get a massage, your current physical condition, medical history, lifestyle and stress level. The massage therapist may ask you about your health goals and what you hope the massage will do to help you achieve those goals.

For a full-body massage, you will be asked to remove clothing to your level of comfort. Undressing takes place in private, and a sheet, towel or gown is provided for draping. The therapist will undrape only the part of your body being massaged, ensuring that your modesty is respected at all times. Your massage, which can last from 30 to 90 minutes, will take place in a comfortable atmosphere and on a cushioned table. You should expect a peaceful, relaxing experience.

Although aromatherapy is an unregulated practice in the U.S., massage therapy (including aromatherapeutic massage) is currently regulated in 30 states and the District of Columbia. The remaining states leave any regulation of massage therapy to local municipalities. Statewide regulation of massage therapists may determine if your insurance directly covers massage by a massage therapist.

Osteopathy

Doctors of osteopathy (D.O.s) truly practice integrative medicine by combining conventional medical practices with osteopathic manipulation, physical therapy and education about healthful posture and body positioning. But the real difference between an M.D and a D.O. is that osteopaths hold to the common sense principle that a patient's history of illnesses and physical traumas are written into the body's structure. It is the osteopath's highly developed sense of touch that allows the physician to feel the patient's "living anatomy" (i.e. flow of fluids, motion of tissues and structural make-up). In fact, a D.O. can even detect physical problems that fail to appear on an X-ray.

Unlike a conventional doctor, the osteopath's job is to "set" the body up

HEART SMART TIP

Osteopathy may relieve angina since tensions in the neck, shoulders and back can serve to aggravate chest pain.

to heal itself. To restore this normal function, the osteopath gently applies a precise amount of force to promote movement of the bodily fluids, eliminate dysfunction in the motion of the tissues, and release compressed bones and joints. In addition, the areas being treated require proper positioning to assist the body's ability to regain normal tissue function.

Osteopathic physicians not only understand that all the body's systems are interconnected, but how each one affects the others. They focus special attention on the musculoskeletal system, which reflects and influences the condition of all other body systems. This system of bones and muscles makes up about two-thirds of the body's mass, and a routine part of the osteopathic patient examination is a careful evaluation of these important structures.

Bringing the body into a state of homeostasis (the process of continual adjustments the body makes to keep itself in a stable condition and function to the best of its ability), an osteopath can also improve the way the heart functions. For example, in the blood there must be a precise quantity of dissolved oxygen within maximum and minimum levels in order for all the body tissues to work. The body is constantly readjusting to maintain this balance.

What To Expect

You may be surprised to find that going to see an osteopath is similar to a conventional doctor visit. Along with a complete physical examination, you may also undergo diagnostic tests, including blood and urine tests and X-rays. But, unlike an allopathic physician, a D.O. will also look at your body structure to assess posture, spine, balance, tendons and ligaments.

An osteopath undergoes as much training as an M.D. (except osteopathy emphasizes preventive medicine and training in musculoskeletal manipulation and hands-on assessment techniques). Because of this, they are licensed in all states as full physicians and can prescribe drugs and perform surgery.

Reflexology

Reflexology is a natural healing art based on the principle that there are reflexes in the hands and feet that correspond to every part of the body. Through application of pressure on these reflexes, reflexology relieves tension, improves circulation and promotes the natural function of the related areas of the body.

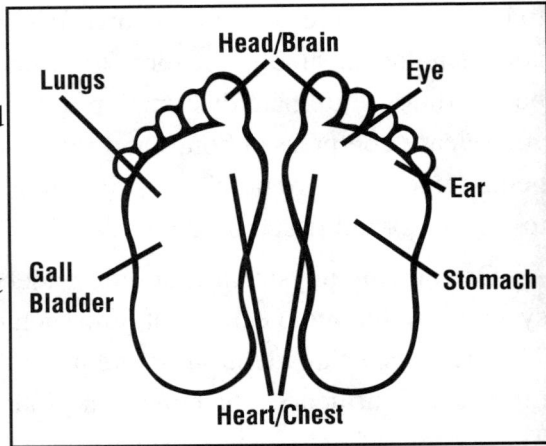

Although reflexology does not diagnose or treat specific ailments by definition, it has proven highly successful over time to relieve symptoms or ease pain or discomfort that have manifested themselves physically in the body - either as a result of stress, trauma or disease.

Studies have shown that reflexology can reduce stress and its related problems – an important benefit if you suffer from heart disease – by positively affecting the central nervous system. For example, massaging the appropriate areas in the feet is thought to help reduce raised blood pressure and relieve angina. It also increases circulation.

What To Expect

You will lie on your back on a massage table, face up, with your shoes and socks removed. To make your feet and ankles more accessible to the reflexologist, it's a good idea to wear shorts or sweat pants. You will be made comfortable with a blanket and soft music. Healing oils may be applied before or after session.

Aromatherapy may be diffused in the room to aid relaxation

and increase your senses. Although most of the treatment is focused on the feet, the last ten minutes is concentrated on the hands. While pain isn't something normally experienced, tender spots will indicate areas that need extra attention. Pressure, as in regular massage, should be "strong but not uncomfortable."

When you are through you should feel relaxed and

Safety Alert!

Ensure that you go to a qualified practitioner and make sure you tell your reflexologist about any drugs you are taking. Most practitioners believe that reflexology can interfere with the effects of some medications.

Reflexology should be used only as an adjunct to medical treatment and not as a replacement for it.

invigorated. You are then sent on your way with the expectation that you will have some internal cleansing take place. It is recommended that you drink plenty of water for the rest of the day to facilitate this cleansing process.

Regular treatments last approximately one hour. For preventative maintenance, treatments are recommended once or twice per month (more if desired). For more serious health problems, treatments can be done much more frequently.

REMEMBER . . .

➤ Complimentary and alternative medicine (CAM) offers a variety of therapies that help prevent and treat heart disease. Along with their beneficial effects on the heart, many of these therapies also reduce stress.

➤ Acupuncture, which uses specialized needles to stimulate "chi," is effective for reducing chest pain and high blood pressure. It may also help treat ischemia and regulate the heart rate.

➤ Like acupuncture, acupressure is a safe and effective way to lower blood pressure and heart rate.

➤ Aromatherapeutic massage combines the medicinal properties of essential oils with healing touch.

➤ Studies show that aromatherapeutic massage can lower blood pressure and increase circulation. It may also benefit people with atherosclerosis.

➤ Never use undiluted oils and do a patch test when using new oils.

➤ Osteopathic physicians combine conventional medicine with physical manipulation to treat the whole person and help the body heal itself.

➤ Reflexology is based on the principal that reflex points on the feet and hands correspond to every part of the body. By manipulating the proper points, a reflexologist can increase circulation and lower stress. It may also reduce blood pressure and chest pain.

About the Author

A practicing physician since 1969, Dr. Robert D. Willix, Jr.'s pioneering work in preventative and integrative health care has earned him national recognition as a healer, teacher, speaker and author.

Dr. Willix graduated Alpha Omega Alpha from the University of Missouri Medical School, and did his Internship and Residency in cardiac surgery at the University of Michigan in Ann Arbor, Michigan. As the first board-certified cardiac surgeon in South Dakota, Dr. Willix started the state's first open-heart surgery program, performed thousands of coronary bypass operations and taught at the University of South Dakota Medical School. In 1981, he was recruited to South Florida as Medical Director for Cardiac Rehabilitation and Human Performance for a major hospital district.

Yet his study of the mind-body connection and the body's innate ability to heal itself inspired him to look at his career in an entirely new way. Seeing the potential of wellness-oriented, non-surgical integrative medicine, he left the surgical suite forever and devoted his practice to making - and keeping - his patients healthy. Convinced that bypass surgery was a "waste of time" if it wasn't accompanied by lifestyle changes, Dr. Willix began a cardiac rehabilitation program based on nutrition, exercise and natural healing traditions. In 1993, he expanded his practice to include Ayurvedic medicine, an ancient form of natural medicine presently being studied by the National Institute of Health's division of Alternative Medicine.

In the 80's, Dr. Willix developed and studied preventive medicine programs, in the 90's, Alternative Medicine approaches of Ayurveda, homeopathy, acupuncture, and other forms of mind-body and herbal systems of healing. At the turn of the Century

2000, Dr. Willix expanded his studies to include the ancient energetic healing technique of the Andean Shaman (the Inka).

Dr. Willix now includes Preventive Medicine, Integrative Medicine, and Shamanic Medicine into his medical repertoire. He believes healing and health require "balance of the body, mind, and spirit."

In addition to his private practice in Boca Raton, Florida, Dr. Willix is the author of *Age PROOFING - 7 Simple Steps to Super Vitality at Any Age, Keep Your Miles High and Your Calories Low*, and *Healthy at 100*. A dedicated amateur athlete, he has competed in 14 marathons and 100 triathlons, including the world championship of triathlons: The IRONMAN in Kona, Hawaii in 1984. Most recently, he has begun to pursue competition in competitive bicycle races-The Criterium Series of United States Cycling Federation.

Appendix I

RESOURCES

Acupressure Institute
1533 Shattuck Avenue
Berkeley, CA 94709
Phone: (510) 845-1059
Website: www.acupressure.com
The Acupressure Institute offers career training, educational material and referrals to certified acupressurists around the country.

American Academy of Medical Acupuncture
4929 Wilshire Blvd., Ste. 428
Los Angeles, CA 90010
Office: (323)937-5514
Fax: (323)937-0959
Website: www.medicalacupuncture.org
This professional organization offers a wealth of information on acupuncture, including research, articles and an online journal. Consumers can also get referrals to licensed acupuncturists in their area.

American Association of Naturopathic Physicians
3201 New Mexico Avenue, NW Suite 350
Washington, DC 20016
Toll free: 1 (866) 538-2267
Local: (202) 895-1392
Fax: (202) 274-1992
Website: www.naturopathic.org
Naturopathic medicine includes therapeutic nutrition, botanical medicine, homeopathy, natural childbirth, classical Chinese medicine, hydrotherapy, naturopathic manipulative therapy,

pharmacology and minor surgery. This professional organization publishes a listing of naturopathic physicians on its website.

American Botanical Council

P.O. Box 144345

Austin, TX 78714

Phone: (512) 926-4900

Fax: (512) 926-2345

Website: www.herbalgram.org

This non-profit educational organization disseminates science-based information on herbal medicine. Its website offers a wide array of books, herb monographs, special reports and computer software.

American College for Advancement in Medicine

23121 Verdugo Drive, Suite 204

Laguna Hills, CA 92653

Phone: (800) 532-3688

Fax: (949) 455-9679

Website: www.acam.org

The American College for Advancement in Medicine is a not-for-profit medical society dedicated to educating physicians and other health care professionals on the latest findings and emerging procedures in preventive/nutritional medicine. Most of its members practice chelation therapy. You can find a practitioner in your area on their website.

American Heart Association

7272 Greenville Ave.

Dallas, TX 75231

(800) 242-8721

Website: www.americanheart.org

The American Heart Association is one of the leading authorities on heart disease and stroke. While the organization primarily focuses on conventional solutions, its website is a good source of information on heart disease. Their website also offers a number of publications and a heart and stroke encyclopedia.

American Osteopathic Association
142 East Ontario St.
Chicago, IL 60611
Phone: (800) 621-1773
Website: www.osteopathic.org
Osteopathic medicine treats the whole person, not simply the symptoms of disease. Practitioners undergo as much training as an M.D. and are required to pass state licensing. However, a doctor of osteopathy (D.O.) receives extra training in the musculoskeletal system. This training provides osteopathic physicians with a better understanding of the ways that an injury or illness in one part of your body can affect another. Along with referrals, this professional group provides an amazing amount of information to consumers.

The Association for Applied Psychophysiology and Biofeedback
10200 W. 44th Avenue, Suite 304
Wheat Ridge, CO 80033-2840
Phone: 1 (800) 477-8892 / (303) 422-8436
Fax: (303) 422-8894
Website: www.aapb.org
E-mail: AAPB@resourcenter.com
This non-profit organization provides a comprehensive explanation of biofeedback through its website and various publications. It also sponsors research and offers referrals to qualified practitioners.

EECP.com
180 Linden Avenue
Westbury, NY 11590
Phone: (800) 455-3327 or (516) 997-4600
Fax: (516) 997-2299
Website: www.eecp.com
This is a website run by Vasomedical, Inc., the company that makes the equipment for EECP, so it is not unbiased. But it does offer an excellent means of finding a center where you can get EECP in your area. Unfortunately, there are fewer than 200 centers which offer EECP, though the number is growing rapidly.

HeartCenterOnline
One South Ocean Boulevard, Suite 201
Boca Raton, FL 33432
FAX: (561) 620-9799
Website: www.heartcenteronline.com
This website is a treasure trove of information on the various aspects of heart disease. It also offers a personalized health tracker.

International Institute of Reflexology
5650 First Ave. North
P.O. Box 12642
St. Petersburg, FL 33733-2642
Phone: (727) 343-4811
Website: www.reflexology-usa.net
Along with referrals, this group provides consumer information and educational workshops, books, charts and videos for practitioners.

The National Association for Holistic Aromatherapy
4509 Interlake Ave N., #233
Seattle, WA 98103-6773
Phone: (888) ASK-NAHA or (206) 547-2164
Fax: (206) 547-2680
Website: www.naha.org
The National Association for Holistic Aromatherapy is an educational, nonprofit organization dedicated to enhancing public awareness of the benefits of true aromatherapy. Along with an extensive list of companies offering pure essential oils, aromatherapy schools and a list of members, the NAHA also publishes the *Aromatherapy Journal.*

National Certification Board for Therapeutic Massage & Bodywork
8201 Greensboro Drive, Suite 300
McLean, VA 22102
Phone: 1 (800) 296-0664 or (703) 610-9015
Fax: (703) 610-9005
E-mail: info@ncbtmb.com
If you are looking for a massage therapist, this group can refer you to a certified practitioner in your area. Along with maintaining a listing of nationally certified massage therapists and reflexologists, the NCBTMB also provides education and certification.

The National Heart, Lung, and Blood Institute
Phone: (301) 592-8573
Fax: (301) 592-8563
Website: www.nhlbi.nih.gov
The NHLBI Health Information Center provides information on a number of health problems, including angina, hypertension, arrhythmia, heart attacks and congestive heart failure. Their website contains interactive tools including a body mass index calculator, a menu planer and a 10-year heart attack risk calculator.

Appendix II

General Medical Terms Relating To Heart Disease

While learning about heart disease and its symptoms, you may find a number of unfamiliar terms. This glossary, adapted from the National Heart, Lung, and Blood Institute of the National Institutes of Health, offers a quick cheat-sheet to help you decipher some of the "medical-speak" you'll come across.

Aneurysms

Small blister-like outpouchings of blood vessel walls. They can rupture, causing bleeding.

Angina

Angina pectoris or angina is a recurring pain or discomfort in the chest. It happens when some part of the heart does not receive enough blood. It can feel like a heaviness, a burning sensation, a discomfort in the left arm or jaw.

Angioplasty/Balloon Angioplasty

A procedure to open clogged arteries. A catheter, positioned in the narrowed coronary artery, has a tiny balloon at its tip. The balloon is inflated and deflated to stretch or break open the narrowing and improve the passage for blood flow. The balloon-tipped catheter is then removed.

Arrhythmia

Arrhythmia or dysrhythmia is a change in the normal heartbeat.

Arteriosclerosis

General term for the thickening and the hardening of arteries. Its development is accelerated by high blood pressure.

Artery

Vessels that carry oxygen-rich blood from the heart to the body. The major arteries of the heart are called the coronary arteries.

Atherosclersosis

A type of arteriosclerosis in which cholesterol, fat and other substances in the blood build up in the walls of arteries. As the process continues, the arteries to the heart may narrow, cutting down the flow of oxygen-rich blood and nutrients to the heart.

Atrial fibrillation

Condition in which the two small upper chambers of the heart, the atria, quiver instead of beating effectively. Although atrial fibrillation is not in itself considered life-threatening, people with it are at an increased risk for blood clots and stroke.

Blood pressure

Blood pressure is the amount of force exerted by the blood against the walls of the arteries. Usually, blood pressure is expressed in two numbers, such as 120/80, and is measured in millimeters of mercury (mm Hg).

Bradycardia

A slower than normal heartbeat.

Bypass Surgery

In a coronary artery bypass operation, a blood vessel, usually taken from the leg or chest, is grafted onto the blocked artery, bypassing the blocked area. If more than one artery is blocked, a bypass can be done on each. The blood can then go around the obstruction to supply the heart with enough blood to relieve chest pain.

C-Reactive protein

A useful biological marker for arterial inflammation. High levels can predict the risk of heart attacks and stroke years before a patient has his or her first coronary event.

Cardiovascular diseases

Diseases of the heart and blood vessel system, such as coronary heart disease, heart attack, high blood pressure, stroke, angina (chest pain), and rheumatic heart disease.

Cerebrovascular diseases

Diseases of the brain and its main blood vessels. In a stroke, for example, the loss of blood flow results in sudden loss of function of part of the brain. Stroke may be caused by a clot (thrombosis) or rupture (hemorrhage) of a blood vessel to the brain.

Cholesterol

A waxy substance produced by the body and taken in with food. The body needs cholesterol for functions such as making hormones. When too much cholesterol circulates in the blood, it leads to atherosclerosis and an increased risk of heart disease. Blood cholesterol refers to the cholesterol circulating in the bloodstream; dietary cholesterol is the cholesterol consumed in food.

Congestive heart failure (CHF)

Also called heart failure. A serious condition in which the heart is unable to pump enough blood to supply the body's needs. CHF occurs when excess fluid starts to leak into the lungs, causing breathing difficulty, fatigue and weakness, and sleeping problems. High blood pressure is the number one risk factor for CHF.

Coronary heart disease (CHD)

The most common form of heart disease. This type of heart disease is caused by a narrowing of the coronary arteries that feed the heart, which results in not enough oxygen-carrying blood reaching the heart.

Diastolic blood pressure

The second or bottom number in a blood pressure reading. Diastolic blood pressure is the minimum pressure that remains within the artery when the heart is at rest.

Endocarditis

Bacterial endocarditis occurs when bacteria in the blood stream lands on abnormal heart valves or other damaged heart tissue.

Fibrinogen

A protein molecule synthesized by the liver which is essential for normal blood clotting. High levels can increase clotting and the risk of heart disease

Heart disease

Diseases of the heart. These include conditions that affect the heart's valves and muscle.

Heart failure

Also called congestive heart failure. A serious condition in which the heart is unable to pump enough blood to supply the body's needs. CHF occurs when excess fluid starts to leak into the lungs, causing breathing difficulty, fatigue and weakness, and sleeping problems. High blood pressure is the number one risk factor for CHF.

High blood pressure

When blood pressure stays above normal levels over a period of time.

Homocystine

An amino acid produced by the body. Elevated levels of homocystine in the blood can damage blood vessels and disrupt normal blood clotting, increasing the risk of heart attack, stroke, and peripheral vascular disease.

Hypertension

The medical term for high blood pressure (blood pressure reading of 140/90 mm Hg or higher).

Ischemic

Refers to the state of not having enough blood flow.

Isolated systolic hypertension (ISH)

A condition in older adults in which only the systolic blood pressure is high (systolic at or above 140 mm Hg and diastolic under 90 mm Hg). ISH is the most common form of high blood pressure for older Americans.

Lipids

Fatty substances, including cholesterol and triglycerides, that are present in blood and body tissues.

Lipoprotein Profile

A blood test that measures cholesterol numbers, usually done after a 9-12 hour fast. The test gives information about total cholesterol, LDL (bad) cholesterol, HDL (good) cholesterol and triglycerides.

Lipoproteins

Protein-coated packages that carry fat and cholesterol through the bloodstream.

mm Hg

Abbreviation for millimeters of mercury. It is used to express measures of blood pressure. It refers to the height to which the pressure in your blood vessels would push a column of mercury.

Murmur

Heart murmurs are sounds made as the blood moves through the heart.

Myocardial Infarction

When the heart does not get enough blood flow and the heart muscle dies. Also known as a heart attack.

Pacemaker

A pacemaker is a small battery-operated electronic device that is used to help the heart beat regularly. Can be used in the treatment of arrhythmia.

PTCA - Percutaneous Transluminal Coronary Angioplasty

A procedure to open clogged arteries. A catheter, positioned in the narrowed coronary artery, has a tiny balloon at its tip. The balloon is inflated and deflated to stretch or break open the narrowing and improve the passage for blood flow. The balloon-tipped catheter is then removed.

Risk factors

Risk factors are traits or habits that make a person more likely to develop a disease. Some risk factors can be controlled, while others - such as age and gender - cannot be. Controllable risk factors for hypertension include cigarette smoking, high blood pressure, high blood cholesterol, overweight or obesity.

Stenosis

Stenosis or narrowing can happen in heart disease to a valve when the valve is stiff and can't open all the way. The result is that the heart must work harder to move blood.

Stent

A stent is a wire mesh tube that's permanently inserted into an artery to help keep it from closing up again. Stents can be used along with angioplasty to help keep an artery open following a heart attack.

Stroke

Sudden loss of function of part of the brain because of loss of blood flow. Stroke may be caused by a clot (thrombosis) or rupture (hemorrhage) of a blood vessel to the brain.

Systolic blood pressure

The first or top number in a blood pressure reading. The maximum pressure produced as the heart contracts and blood begins to flow. As systolic pressure rises, especially reaching or passing 140, so does the risk of getting heart disease.

Tachycardia

A rapid heartbeat.

Thrombus

A blood clot.

Triglycerides

Lipids carried through the bloodstream to tissues. Most of the body's fat tissue is in the form of triglycerides, stored for use as energy. Triglycerides are obtained primarily from fat in foods.

Unstable Angina

Chest pain that occurs at rest; new onset of pain with exertion; or pain that has accelerated (i.e., more frequent, longer in duration, or lower in threshold).

Vascular

A term to describe blood vessels.

Veins

Vessels that carry blood from the body to the heart.

SELECTED REFERENCES
Chapter 1

"Cigarettes: What the warning label doesn't tell you." American Council on Science and Health, 1996.

"Diabetes Doubles Heart Disease Death Risk; Diabetes Control Approach May Effect Outcomes." DukeMed News. 21 Mar 2001.

Fu T, et al. "Macrophage uptake of low-density lipoprotein bound to aggregated C-reactive protein: possible mechanism of foam-cell formation in atherosclerotic lesions." *Biochemical Journal*. 2002; 366:195-201.

NJ Wald, et al. "Homocystine and ischaemic heart disease: results of a prospective study with implications regarding prevention." *Archives of Internal Medicine*. 1998;158: 862-7.

O Nygård JE, et al. "Plasma homocystine and mortality in patients with coronary artery disease." *New England Journal of Medicine*. 1997;337: 230-6.

Ridker PM, et al. "Inflammation, aspirin, and the risk of cardiovascular disease in apparently healthy men." *New England Journal of Medicine*. 1997;336:973-979.

"Risk Factors and Coronary Heart Disease." American Heart Association. AHA/ACC Scientific Statement: Assessment of Cardiovascular Risk by Use of Multiple-Risk-Factor Assessment Equations, #71-0177." *Circulation*. 1999;100:1481-1492.

"Smoking and Heart Disease." Methodist Health Care System. Houston, TX. 2003.

Yip J, et al. "Resistance to insulin-mediated glucose disposal as a predictor of cardiovascular disease." *Journal of Clinical Endocrinology & Metabolism.* 1998;83:2773-2776.

Chapter 2

"Heart Disease and Stroke Statistics: 2003 Update." American Heart Association.

"Leading Causes of Death, 2000." Statistical Fact Sheet. American Heart Association.

Chapter 3

American College of Chest Physicians 69th annual international scientific assembly, Orlando, Fla., Oct. 25-30, 2003.

Abstract 1494. *Circulation.* 2002; SII, 106:19.

Griffith LS. "Changes in intrinsic coronary circulation and segmental ventricular motion after saphenous vein coronary bypass graft surgery." *New England Journal of Medicine.* 1973;288:589.

Hung J. "Aspirin for cardiovascular disease prevention." *Medical Journal of Australia.* 2003;179:147-152.

Kent SM, et al. "Effect of atorvastatin and pravastatin on serum C-reactive protein." *American Heart Journal.* 2003;145:e8.

Koster R, et al. "Nickel and molybdenum contact allergies in patients with coronary in-stent restenosis." *Lancet.* 2000;356:1895-1897.

Maron DJ. "Percutaneous coronary intervention versus medical therapy for coronary heart disease." *Current Atherosclerosis Report*. 2000;2:290-296.

Meade TW, et al. "Determination of who may derive most benefit from aspirin in primary prevention: subgroup results from a randomised controlled trial." *British Medical Journal*. 2000;321:13-17.

Newman MF, et al. "Longitudinal assessment of neurocognitive function after coronary-artery bypass surgery." *New England Journal of Medicine*. 2001;344:395-402.

Pahor M, et al. "Calcium channel blockade and incidence of cancer in aged populations." *Lancet*. 1996;348:493-497.

Pahor M, et al. "Health outcomes associated with calcium antagonists compared with other first-line antihypertensive therapies: a met-analysis of randomized controlled trials." *Lancet*. 2000;356:1949-1954.

Psaty BM, et al. "The risk of myocardial infarction associated with antihypertensive drug therapies." *Journal of the American Medical Association*. 1995;274:620-625.

Seides SF. "Coronary problems after bypass surgery." *New England Journal of Medicine*. 1978;298:1213-1217.

Chapter 4

Albert CM, et al. "Fish consumption and risk of sudden cardiac death." *Journal of the American Medical Association*. 1998;279:23-28.

Albert CM, et al. "Nut consumption and decreased risk of sudden cardiac death in the Physicians' Health Study." *Archives of Internal Medicine*. 2002;162:1382-1387.

Axelrod L, et al. "Effects of a small quantity of omega-3 fatty acids on cardiovascular risk factors in NIDDM. A randomized, prospective, double-blind, controlled study." *Diabetes Care*. 1994;17:37-44.

Bursill C, et al. "Green tea upregulates the low-density lipoprotein receptor through the sterol-regulated element binding Protein in HepG2 liver cells." *Journal of Agricultural and Food Chemistry*. 2001;49:5639-5645.

Carluccio MA, "Olive oil and red wine antioxidant polyphenols inhibit endothelial activation: antiatherogenic properties of mediterranean diet phytochemicals." *Arteriosclerosis, Thrombosis and Vascular Biology*. 2003; 23:622-629.

Davies MJ, et al. "Black Tea Consumption Reduces Total and LDL Cholesterol in Mildly Hypercholesterolemic Adults." *Journal of Nutrition*. 2003;133:3298S-3302S.

Deepak PV, et al. "Use of antioxidant vitamins for the prevention of cardiovascular disease: meta-analysis of randomised trials." *Lancet*. 2003; 361:2017-2023.

Devaraj S, et al. "Alpha tocopherol supplementation decreases serum C-reactive protein and monocyte interleukin-6 levels in normal volunteers and type 2 diabetic patients." *Free Radical Biology & Medicine*. 2000; 29:790-792.

Goodnight SH, et al. "The effects of dietary omega 3 fatty acids on platelet composition and function in man: a prospective, controlled study." *Blood.* 1981;58:880-885.

He J, et al. "Dietary sodium intake and subsequent risk of cardiovascular disease in overweight adults." *Journal of the American Medical Association.* 1999;282:2027-2034.

Hu FB, et al. "Dietary fat and coronary heart disease: a comparison of approaches for adjusting for total energy intake and modeling repeated dietary measurements." *American Journal of Epidemiology.* 1999; 149:531-540.

Katan MB. "Trans fatty acids and plasma lipoproteins." *Nutrition Reviews.* 2000; 58:188-91.

Kris-Etherton PM, et al. "The effects of nuts on coronary heart disease risk." *Nutrition Review.* 2001;59:103-111.

Kritchevsky SB. "Beta-carotene, carotenoids and the prevention of coronary heart disease." *Journal of Nutrition.* 1999;129:5-8.

Law MR, Morris JK. "By how much does fruit and vegetable consumption reduce the risk of ischaemic heart disease?" *European Journal of Clinical Nutrition.* 1998;52:549-56.

Lee CD, et al. "Cardiorespiratory fitness, body composition, and all-cause and cardiovascular disease mortality in men." *American Journal of Clinical Nutrition.* 1999;69:373–80.

Lemaitre, Rozenn N., et al. "Cell membrane trans-fatty acids and the risk of primary cardiac arrest." *Circulation.* 2002;105:697-701.

Liu S, et al. "A prospective study of dietary fiber intake and risk of cardiovascular disease among women." *Journal of the American College of Cardiology*. 2002;39:49-56.

Liu S, et al. "Relation between changes in intakes of dietary fiber and grain products and changes in weight and development of obesity among middle-aged women." *American Journal of Clinical Nutrition*. 2003;78: 920-927.

Madsen T, et al. "C-reactive protein, dietary n-3 fatty acids, and the extent of coronary artery disease." *American Journal of Cardiology*. 2001;88:1139-1142.

Palace VP, et al. "Antioxidant potentials of vitamin A and carotenoids and their relevance to heart disease." *Free Radical Biology and Medicine*. 1999;26:746-761.

"PCBs in Farmed Salmon: Factory Methods, Unnatural Results." Environmental Working Group. 30 Jul 2003. Available at www.egw.org.

Pischon T, et al. "Habitual dietary intake of n-3 and n-6 fatty acids in relation to inflammatory markers among US men and women." *Circulation*. 2003 Jul 15;108(2):155-160.

Pietinen P, et al. "Intake of dietary fiber and risk of coronary heart disease in a cohort of Finnish men. The Alpha-Tocopherol, Beta-Carotene Cancer Prevention Study." *Circulation*. 1996;94:2720-2427.

Sacks FM, et al. "Effects on blood pressure of reduced dietary sodium and the Dietary Approaches to Stop Hypertension

(DASH) diet. DASH-Sodium Collaborative Research Group."
New England Journal of Medicine. 2001;344:3-10.

Strandhagen E, et al. "High fruit intake may reduce mortality
among middle-aged and elderly men. The Study of Men Born in
1913." *European Journal of Clinical Nutrition.* 2000;54:337-341.

Tchernof A, et al. "Weight loss reduces C-reactive protein levels
in obese postmenopausal women." *Circulation.* 2002;105:564-
569.

Torres, Isabel C., et al. "Study of the effects of dietary fish intake
on serum lipids and lipoproteins in two populations with different
dietary habits." *British Journal of Nutrition.* 2000;83:371-379.

Tribble D, "Antioxidant consumption and risk of coronary heart
disease: emphasis on vitamin C, vitamin E, and beta-carotene."
Circulation. 1999; 99:591-595.

Trichopoulou A, et al. "Adherence to a Mediterranean diet and
survival in a Greek population." *New England Journal of
Medicine.* 2003; 348:2599-2608.

Tuck KL, et al. "Major phenolic compounds in olive oil:
metabolism and health effects." *Journal of Nutrition and
Biochemistry.* 2002; 13:636-644.

Weinberger MH, et al. "Salt sensitivity, pulse pressure, and death
in normal and hypertensive humans." *Hypertension.* 2001;37:429-
32.

Chapter 5

Blair SN, et al. "Influences of cardiorespiratory fitness and other precursors on cardiovascular disease and all-cause mortality in men and women ." *Journal of the American Medical Association.* 1996;276:205-210.

Church TS, et al. "Association between cardiorespiratory fitness and C-reactive protein in men." *Arteriosclerosis, Thrombosis, and Vascular Biology.* 2002;22:1869.

Hakim, A, et al. "Effects of walking on coronary heart disease in elderly men: The Honolulu Heart Program." *Circulation.* 1999;100: 9-13.

Hambrecht R, et al. "Effects of exercise training on left ventricular function and peripheral resistance in patients with chronic heart failure: A randomized trial." *Journal of the American Medical Association.* 2000;283:3095-3101.

Iwasaki K, et al. "Dose-response relationship of the cardiovascular adaptation to endurance training in healthy adults: how much training for what benefit?" *Journal of Applied Physiology.* 2003;95:1575-1583.

Kraemer WJ, et al. "Resistance training for health and performance." *Current Sports Medicine Reports.* 2002;1:165-171.

Kraus, WE, et al. "Effects of the Amount and Intensity of Exercise on Plasma Lipoproteins." *New England Journal of Medicine.* 2002; 347:1483-1492.

Lemaitre RN, et al. "Leisure-time physical activity and the risk of nonfatal myocardial infarction in postmenopausal women." *Archives of Internal Medicine.* 1995;155:2302-2308.

Leo I, et al. "Physical activity and coronary heart disease in women: is "no pain, no gain" passé?" *Journal of the American Medical Association.* 2001;285:1447-1454.

Manson JE et al. "A prospective study of walking as compared with vigorous exercise in the prevention of coronary heart disease in women." *New England Journal of Medicine.* 1999;341:650-658.

McGuire DK, et al. "A 30-year follow-up of the Dallas Bedrest and Training Study: II. Effect of age on cardiovascular adaptation to exercise training." *Circulation.* 2001;104:1358-1366.

Roberts CK, et al. "Effect of diet and exercise intervention on blood pressure, insulin, oxidative stress, and nitric oxide availability." *Circulation.* 2002;106:2530-2532.

Stone MH, et al. "Health and performance-related potential of resistance training." *Sports Medicine.* 1991;11:210-231.

Toskovic NN, et al. "The effect of experience and gender on cardiovascular and metabolic responses with dynamic Tae Kwon Do exercise." *Journal of Strength Conditioning Research.* 2002;16:278-285.

Chapter 6

Ayas NT, et al. "A prospective study of sleep duration and coronary heart disease in women." *Archives of Internal Medicine.* 2003;163: 205-209.

Blumenthal JA, et al. "Usefulness of psychosocial treatment of mental stress-induced myocardial ischemia in men." *American Journal of Cardiology.* 2002;89:164-168.

Kanagala R, et al. "Obstructive sleep apnea and the recurrence of atrial fibrillation." *Circulation.* 2003;107:2589-2594.

Katz J, et al. "Association Between Periodontal Pockets and Elevated Cholesterol and Low Density Lipoprotein Cholesterol Levels." *Journal of Periodontology.* 2002;73:494-500.

Landmark K. "Smoking and coronary heart disease." *Tidsskrift for den Norske laegeforening.* 2001;121:1710-1712.

Law MR, et al. "Environmental tobacco smoke and ischemic heart disease." *Progress in Cardiovascular Diseases.* 2003;46:31-38.

Linden W, et al. "Individualized stress management for primary hypertension: a randomized trial." *Archives of Internal Medicine.* 2001;161:1071-1080.

Lusardi P, et al. "Effects of insufficient sleep on blood pressure in hypertensive patients: a 24-h study." *American Journal of Hypertension.* 1999;12:63-68.

Plante GE. "Vascular response to stress in health and disease." *Metabolism.* 2002; 51: 25-30.

Richards JC, et al. "Serum lipids and their relationships with hostility and angry affect and behaviors in men." *Health Psychology.* 2000;19:393-398.

Rutledge T, et al. "Psychosocial variables are associated with atherosclerosis risk factors among women with chest pain: the WISE study." *Psychosomatic Medicine.* 2001;63:282-288.

Stoney CM, et al. "Acute psychological stress reduces plasma triglyceride clearance." *Psychophysiology.* 2002;39:80-85.

Chapter 7

Adler A, Holub B. "Effect of garlic and fish-oil supplementation on serum lipid and lipoprotein concentrations in hypercholesterolemic men." *American Journal of Clinical Nutrition.* 1997;65:445-450.

Anand I, et al. "Acute and chronic effect of propionyl-L-carnitine on the hemodynamics, exercise capacity and hormones of patients with congestive heart failure." *Cardiovascular Drugs and Therapy.* 1998; 12:291-299.

Arruzazabala ML, et al. "Comparative study of policosanol, aspirin and the combination therapy policosanol-aspirin on platelet aggregation in healthy volunteers." *Pharmacological Research.* 1997;36:293–297.

Bostick RM, et al. "Relation of calcium, vitamin D and dairy food intake to ischemic heart disease mortality among postmenopausal women." *American Journal of Epidemiology.* 1999;149:151-161.

Digiesi V, et al. "The benefits of L-carnitine in essential arterial hypertension." *Minerva Medica.* 1989;80:227-231.

Douglas D. "Magnesium in diet may alter heart disease risk." *Reuters.* 10 October 2003.

Enstrom JE, et al. "Vitamin C intake and mortality among a sample of the United States population." *Epidemiology.* 1992;3:194-202.

Franconi F. "Plasma and platelet taurine are reduced in subjects with insulin-dependent diabetes mellitus: Effects of taurine supplementation," *American Journal of Clinical Nutrition.* 1995; 61:1115-1119.

Friedberg C, et al. "Fish oil and glycemic control in diabetes. A meta-analysis." *Diabetes Care.* 1998;21:494-500.

Galloe A, et al. "Influence of oral magnesium supplementation on cardiac events among survivors of an acute myocardial infarction." *British Medical Journal.* 1993;307:585–587.

Gouni-Berthold I, Berthold HK. "Policosanol: clinical pharmacology and therapeutic significance of a new lipid-lowering agent." *American Heart Journal.* 2002;143:356-365.

Hu, Frank B., et al. "Fish and long-chain omega-3 fatty acid intake and risk of coronary heart disease and total mortality in diabetic women." *Circulation.* 2003;107:1852-1857.

Kawano Y, et al. "Effects of magnesium supplementation in hypertensive patients: assessment by office, home, and ambulatory blood pressures." *Hypertension.* 1998;32:260-265.

Kardinaal AF, et al. "Association between beta-carotene and acute myocardial infarction depends on polyunsaturated fatty acid status. The EURAMIC Study. European Study on Antioxidants, Myocardial Infarction, and Cancer of the Breast." *Arteriosclerosis, Thrombosis and Vascular Biology.* 1995;15:726-732.

Kohls KJ, et al. "Serum lipid levels of humans given arginine, lysine and tryptophan supplements without food." *Nutrition Reports International.* 1987;35:5-13.

Luo, Jing, et al. "Moderate intake of n-3 fatty acids for 2 months has no detrimental effect on glucose metabolism and could ameliorate the lipid profile in type 2 diabetic men." Diabetes Care. 1998;21:717-724.

Menendez R, et al. "Policosanol modulates HMG-CoA reductase activity in cultured fibroblasts." *Archives of Medical Research.* 2001;32:8-12.

Mancini M, et al. "Controlled study on the therapeutic efficacy of propionyl-L-carnitine in patients with congestive heart failure." *Arzneimittelforschung.* 1992;42:1101-1104.

Matsushita, K. et al, "Nitric Oxide Regulates Exocytosis by S-Nitrosylation of N-ethylmaleimide-Sensitive Factor," *Cell.* 2003;115: 1-20.

Mirkin A, et al. "Efficacy and tolerability of policosanol in hypercholesterolemic postmenopausal women." *International Journal of Clinical Pharmacological Research.* 2001;21:31–41.

Miyazaki Y, et al. "Relationship of dietary intake of fish and non-fish selenium to serum lipids in Japanese rural coastal community." *Journal of Trace Elements in Medicine and Biology.* 2002;16:83-90.

Moore JA, et al. "Selenium concentrations in plasma of patients with arteriographically defined coronary atherosclerosis." *Clinical Chemistry.* 1984;30:1171-1173.

Nozue T, et al. "Magnesium status, serum HDL cholesterol, and apolipoprotein A-1 levels." *Journal of Pediatric Gastroenterology and Nutrition.* 1995;20:316–318.

Park T; Lee K. "Dietary taurine supplementation reduces plasma and liver cholesterol and triglyceride levels in rats fed a high-cholesterol or a cholesterol-free diet." *Advances in Experimental Medicine and Biology.* 1998;442:319-25.

Prat H, et al. "Comparative effects of policosanol and two HMG-CoA reductase inhibitors on type II hypercholesterolemia." *Revista Medica de Chile.* 1999;127:286-294.

Reid IR, et al. "Effects of calcium supplementation on serum lipid concentrations in normal older women: a randomized controlled trial." *American Journal of Medicine.* 2002;112: 343-347.

Rimm EB, et al. "Vitamin E consumption and the risk of coronary heart disease in men." *New England Journal of Medicine.* 1993;337:1.

Rissanen T, et al. "Lycopene, atherosclerosis and coronary heart disease." *Experiments in Biology and Medicine.* 2002;227:900-907.

Selhub J. "Homocystine metabolism". *Annual Review of Nutrition.* 1999;19:217-46.

Sesso HD, et al. "Plasma lycopene, other carotenoids, and retinol and the risk of cardiovascular disease in women." *American Journal of Clinical Nutrition.* 2004;79:47-53.

Singh RB; Niaz MA. "Serum concentration of lipoprotein(a) decreases on treatment with hydrosoluble coenzyme Q10 in patients with coronary artery disease: discovery of a new role." *International Journal of Cardiology.* 1999;68:23-29.

Stefanutti C, et al. "Effect of L-carnitine on plasma lipoprotein fatty acids pattern in patients with primary hyperlipoproteinemia." *La Clinica terapeutica.* 1998;149:115–119.

Stephens NG, et al. "Randomised controlled trial of vitamin E in patients with coronary disease: Cambridge Heart Antioxidant Study (CHAOS)." *Lancet.* 1996;347:781–786.

Takagi Y, et al. "Calcium treatment of essential hypertension in elderly patients evaluated by 24 H monitoring." *American Journal of Hypertension.* 1991;4:836-839.

Visioli F. "Protective activity of tomato products on in vivo markers of lipid oxidation." *European Journal of Nutrition.* 2003;42:201-206.

Wagner JD, et al. "Soy Protein With Isoflavones, but not an Isoflavone-Rich Supplement, Improves Arterial Low-Density Lipoprotein Metabolism and Atherogenesis." *Arteriosclerosis, Thrombosis, and Vascular Biology.* 2003;23:2241.

Wang WT, et al. "Effects of L-arginine on the function of platelet aggregation during hepatic ischemia/reperfusion injury." *Zhongguo Wei Zhong Bing Ji Jiu Yi Xue.* 2004;16:49-51.

Wilcken DE, et al. "Homocystinuria—the effects of betaine in the treatment of patients not responsive to pyridoxine." *New England Journal of Medicine.* 1983;309:448-453.

Wolf A, et al. "Dietary L-arginine supplementation normalizes platelet aggregation in hypercholesterolemic humans." *Journal of the American College of Cardiology.* 1997;29:479-85.

Wollin SD, Jones PJ. "Alpha-lipoic acid and cardiovascular disease." *Journal of Nutrition.* 2003;133:3327-3330.

Chapter 8

Al-Othman AA. "Growth and lipid metabolism responses in rats fed different dietary fat sources." *International Journal of Food Science and Nutrition.* 2000;51:159-167.

Benzie IF, et al. "Consumption of green tea causes rapid increase in plasma antioxidant power in humans." *Nutrition and Cancer.* 1999;34:83–87.

Bharani A, et al. "Efficacy of Terminalia arjuna in chronic stable angina: a double-blind, placebo-controlled, crossover study comparing Terminalia arjuna with isosorbide mononitrate." *Indian Heart Journal.* 2002;54:170-175.

Bordia A, et al. "Effect of Garlic on Platelet Aggregation in Humans: A study in Healthy Subjects and Patients with Coronary Artery Disease." *Prostaglandins, Leukotrienes and Essential Fatty Acids.* 1996;55:201-205.

Fuhrman B, et al. "Ginger extract consumption reduces plasma cholesterol, inhibits LDL oxidation and attenuates development of atherosclerosis in atherosclerotic, apolipoprotein E-deficient mice." *Journal of Nutrition.* 2000;130:1124-1131.

Gupta R, et al "Antioxidant and hypocholesterolaemic effects of Terminalia arjuna tree-bark powder: a randomised placebo-controlled trial." *The Journal of the Association of Physicians of India.* 2001; 49:231-235.

Hayek T, et al. "Reduced progression of atherosclerosis in apolipoprotein E-deficient mice following consumption of red wine, or its polyphenols quercetin or catechin, is associated with reduced susceptibility of LDL to oxidation and aggregation." *Arteriosclerosis, Thrombosis and Vascular Biology.* 1997;17:2744-2752.

Heinicke RM, et al. "Effect of Bromelain (Ananase) on Human Platelet Aggregation." *Experientia.* 1972;28:844-845.

Hollman PC, et al. "Catechin intake might explain the inverse relation between tea consumption and ischemic heart disease: The Zutphen Elderly Study." *American Journal of Clinical Nutrition.* 2001;74:227-232.

Howes JB, et al. "The effects of dietary supplementation with isoflavones from red clover on the lipoprotein profiles of postmenopausal women with mild to moderate hypercholesterolemia." *Atherosclerosis.* 2000;152(1):143-147.

Imai K; Nakachi K. "Cross sectional study of effects of drinking green tea on cardiovascular and liver diseases." *British Medical Journal.* 1995;310:693-696.

Koh JH, et al. "Hypocholesterolemic effect of hot-water extract from mycelia of Cordyceps sinensis." *Biological and Pharmaceutical Bulletin.* 2003;26:84-87.

Koch R "Comparative study of Venostasin and Pycnogenol in chronic venous insufficiency." *Phytotherapy Research.* 2002;16:S1-5.

Koscielny J, et al. "The Anti-atherosclerotic Effect of Allium sativum." *Atherosclerosis.* 1999;144:237-249.

Kudolo GB, et al. "Effect of the ingestion of Ginkgo biloba extract on platelet aggregation and urinary prostanoid excretion in healthy and Type 2 diabetic subjects." *Thrombosis Research.* 2002;108:151-160.

Liebson PR, Amsterdam EA. "Prevention of coronary heart disease. Part I: Primary prevention." *Disease-A-Month.* 1999; 45:497-571.

Mei QB, et al. "Antiarrhythmic effects of Cordyceps sinensis." *Zhongguo Zhong Yao Za Zhi.* 1989;14:616-618, 640.

Munday JS, et al. "Daily supplementation with aged garlic extract, but not raw garlic, protects low density lipoprotein against in vitro oxidation." *Atherosclerosis.* 1999;143:399-404.

Nieper H." Effect of bromelain on coronary heart diseases and angina pectoris." *Journal of the International Academy of Preventive Medicine.* 1976;3:62–63.

Nurtjahja-Tjendraputra E, et al. "Effective anti-platelet and COX-1 enzyme inhibitors from pungent constituents of ginger." *Thrombosis Research.* 2003;111:259-265.

Peters H, et al. "Demonstration of the efficacy of ginkgo biloba special extract EGb 761 on intermittent claudication—a placebo-controlled, double-blind multicenter trial." *Vasa: Journal for Vascular Diseases.* 1998;27:106-110.

Pittler MH, et al. "Artichoke leaf extract for treating hypercholesterolaemia." *Cochrane Database System Review.* 2002;(3):CD003335.

Prasanna M. "Hypolipidemic effect of fenugreek: A clinical study." *Indian Journal of Pharmacology.* 2000;32:34–36.

Quettier-Deleu C, et al. "Hawthorn extracts inhibit LDL oxidation." *Pharmazie.* 2003;58:577-581.

Schmidt U, et al. "Efficacy of the Hawthorn (Crataegus) preparation LI 132 in 78 patients with chronic congestive heart failure defined as NYHA functional class II." *Phytomedicine.* 1994;1:17–24.

Sharma RD, et al. "Effect of fenugreek seeds on blood glucose and serum lipids in type I diabetes." *European Journal of Clinical Nutrition.* 1990;44:301-306.

Singh K, et al. "Guggulsterone, a potent hypolipidaemic, prevents oxidation of low density lipoprotein." *Phytotherapy Research.* 1997;11:291–294.

Sowmya P; Rajyalakshmi P. "Hypocholesterolemic effect of germinated fenugreek seeds in human subjects." *Plant Foods for Human Nutrition.* 1999;53:359-365.

Steiner M, et al. "A double-blind crossover study in moderately hypercholesterolemic men that compared the effect of aged garlic extract and placebo administration on blood lipids." *American Journal of Clinical Nutrition.* 1996;64:866-870.

Tauchert M, et al. "Effectiveness of hawthorn extract LI 132 compared with the ACE inhibitor Captopril: Multicenter double-blind study with 132 patients NYHA stage II. " *Munchener medizinische Wochen-schrift.* 1994;132:S27–33.

Tsubono Y, Tsugane S. "Green tea intake in relation to serum lipid levels in middle-aged Japanese men and women." *Annals of Epidemiology.* 1997;7:280–284.

Visioli F, Galli C. "Antiatherogenic components of olive oil." *Current Atherosclerosis Report.* 2001;3:64-67.

Watson RR. "Pycnogenol and cardiovascular health. " *Evidence-Based Integrative Medicine.* 2003;1:27-32.

Yamaguchi Y, et al. "Antioxidant activity of the extracts from fruiting bodies of cultured Cordyceps sinensis." *Phytotherapy Research.* 2000; 14:647-649.

Xu N, Zhang B. "Effect of Cordyceps on Plasma Lipids in Normal, Stressed, and Hyperlipemic Rats." *Abstracts of Chinese Medicines.* 1987;2:317.

Chapter 9

Born, GR, Geurkink, TL "Improved peripheral vascular function with low dose intravenous ethylene diamine tetraacetic acid (EDTA)." *Townsend Letter for Doctors*. July, 1994, #132, 722-726.

Carter JP. "If EDTA chelation therapy is so good, why is it not more widely accepted." *Journal of Advancement in Medicine*. 1989;2:213-226.

Chappell LT, Stahl JP "The correlation between EDTA Chelation therapy and improvement in cardiovascular function: A Meta-Analysis." *Journal of Advancement in Medicine*, 1993, 6: 3, 139-160.

Chappell LT, Stahl JP, Evans R. "EDTA Chelation treatment for vascular disease: A Meta-Analysis using unpublished data." *Journal of Advancement in Medicine*. 1994, 7: 3, 131-142.

Hancke C, Flytie K. "Benefits of EDTA chelation therapy on arteriosclerosis." *Journal of Advancement in Medicine*. 1993;6:161-72.

Kindness G, Frackelton JP. "Effect of EDTA on platelet aggregation in human blood." *Journal of Advancement in Medicine*. 1989;2:519-530.

Lawson WE, Hui JC, Cohn PF. "Long-term prognosis of patients with angina treated with enhanced external counterpulsation: five-year follow-up study." *Clinical Cardiology*. 2000;23:254-258.

Sloth-Nielsen J, et al. "Arteriographic findings in EDTA chelation therapy on peripheral arteriosclerosis." *American Journal of Surgery.* 1991;162:122-5.

Urano H, Ikeda H, Ueno T, et al. "Enhanced external counterpulsation improves exercise tolerance, reduces exercise-induced myocardial ischemia and improves left ventricular diastolic filling in patients with coronary artery disease." *Journal of the American College of Cardiology.* 2001;37:93-99.

Chapter 10

Felhendler D, Lisander B. "Effects of non-invasive stimulation of acupoints on the cardiovascular system." *Complementary Therapies in Medicine.* 1999;7:231-234.

Feng GM; Xing DJ; Sun QX. "Effects of acupuncture on blood pressure, SOD,LPO and five kinds of trace elements to stenosis of renal artery caused hypertension in rats." *Zhongguo Zhong Xi Yi Jie He Za Zhi.* 1994;14:739-741.

Guo W; Ni G. "The effects of acupuncture on blood pressure in different patients." *Journal of Traditional Chinese Medicine.* 2003; 23:49-50.

Sainani, G.S. "Non-drug therapy in prevention and control of hypertension." *The Journal of the Association of Physicians of India.* 51:1001-6.

Shi X, Wang ZP, Liu KX. "Effect of acupuncture on heart rate variability in coronary heart disease patients." *Zhongguo Zhong Xi Yi Jie He Za Zhi.* 1995;15:536-538.